Community Treatment of Drug Misuse

Community Treatment of Drug Misuse
More than Methadone

Second Edition

Nicholas Seivewright

Assisted by Mark Parry

CAMBRIDGE
UNIVERSITY PRESS

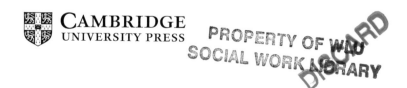

CAMBRIDGE UNIVERSITY PRESS
Cambridge, New York, Melbourne, Madrid, Cape Town,
Singapore, São Paulo, Delhi

Cambridge University Press
The Edinburgh Building, Cambridge CB2 8RU, UK

Published in the United States of America by Cambridge University
Press, New York

www.cambridge.org
Information on this title: www.cambridge.org/9780521691833

First published 2009

Printed in the United Kingdom at the University Press, Cambridge

A catalogue record for this publication is available from the British Library

ISBN 978-0-521-69183-3 paperback

Contents

Preface and acknowledgements

About a decade ago I was extremely grateful to be asked to contribute a volume to a series of social and community psychiatry texts, covering various specialities, by this publisher. The series constituted highly practical guidance with descriptions of local service provision, and mine was to be something similar on treatment of drug misuse. In fact as the planning advanced Cambridge University Press thought it could be a stand-alone text, of value to the many doctors and other clinicians coming into or already established in the field of substance misuse, and so I tried to make the volume comprehensive as well as adding a few flavours of our own services.

Thankfully the combination of quite a thorough review of the evidence for treatments in the various forms of drug misuse plus practical insights has been well-received, and a second edition has been requested. The element of actually describing local services is not as necessary this time, and with the book having been used essentially as a textbook by psychiatrists, primary care physicians and multidisciplinary team workers I wanted to make it definitely function in that regard, therefore requiring an even more detailed review of current literature. To aid with this I knew just the person to recruit to assist, Mark Parry, himself also a consultant psychiatrist in addictions, who is highly expert at searching literature databases and could cut them down to manageable proportions containing the most relevant papers. I could not have done the project in anything like its present form without Mark, who has worked extremely conscientiously over a long period to not only provide the material but give me an additional, expert perspective on clinical aspects. Mark previously trained as a general practitioner, and I hope that he will soon be able to publish what will be very well-informed articles on treatment in primary care and other fields in which he has extensive knowledge, such as managing addicts with painful conditions, as he would provide much more detail than I have been able to do in the relatively short sections in this deliberately wide-ranging text.

Mark's employers have been very understanding in allowing him to work with me on this project, with both of us being full-time doctors in the UK's National Health Service rather than in academic positions. We thank the Berkshire Healthcare NHS Foundation Trust for approving the relevant study leave, and also Mark's local treatment team, the Drug and Alcohol Specialist Service. Finally regarding his work, Mark is extremely grateful to his wife Nilmala and daughter Sarah for their patience and support during the very long hours spent on the project. Similarly I would like to thank my wife Helen and children Paula and Richard, who have known how much I wanted to write this book, and have put up with the strange sight of me working at previously unknown times of day and night!

At the time of the first edition I chose the sub-title 'More than Methadone' because drug services in the UK and elsewhere were needing to broaden their horizons in response to various factors, including a great influx of relatively early-stage heroin users, the rise of cocaine misuse for which substitution therapy is not recommended, a more general concern about non-opiate misusers being neglected even for counselling therapies, and the high-profile publicity regarding alternative maintenance treatments such as diamorphine itself. In fact there has been another major development which is exactly on the theme of that strapline, which is of course buprenorphine as the most direct alternative treatment to methadone in large proportions of heroin users, and there is much more information on the two main preparations containing that drug in this edition. Other subjects more emphasized here are many aspects of so-called 'dual diagnosis' and the liaison and treatments necessary in managing special patient groups, while throughout the text we have made a point of finding up-to-date papers to refer to, and describing the developments which have occurred in relation to the main treatments we describe. We hope therefore that this updated version will be very useful for clinicians from the various disciplines who are involved at the 'sharp end' of delivering services. The way in which I have often found myself describing the book is that if a doctor, nurse or other worker had a clinic to do in an afternoon and they read some relevant parts of the book in the morning, then that would actually be of direct use to them when doing their work, and I have attempted to stick to this principle once again.

In the first edition I expressed my thanks to the many specialists, academics and colleagues in general who had helped me in the earlier stages in my career, in my psychiatric training in Nottingham, the first consultant post and then senior lectureship which I had in Manchester, and more recently those who had worked with me to set up treatment services from a very low starting point in the city of Sheffield. I remain indebted to them all, and it was very kind of Professor John Strang to previously write a Foreword, as he is rightly admired across the world for his commitment to the speciality of drug misuse treatment and his marvellous combination of academic ability and true grasp of clinical realities. Of those who encouraged me at an earlier stage I am most grateful of all to Dr Philip McLean, consultant in addictions in Nottingham, UK, who supervised my first attachment in the field as a junior doctor and who ran the kind of service for his patients that inspired me – and several contemporary colleagues – to join in.

With this second edition, my most important acknowledgement, alongside that to Mark Parry, is to the other person without whom I literally could not have produced the book, my secretary Charlotte Hague. In addition to all her other roles within our service, coordinating staff and assisting with my duties to the Health Service, the General Medical Council and the family courts, she has typed endless drafts of the book and lists of references with unfailing good humour, and I am extremely grateful to her. I also pay tribute to the marvellous staff of the two substance misuse services where I work in Sheffield and North Nottinghamshire, who are expertly led by Sarah Crookes, Giz Sangha, Paul Reeves, Chris Wood, Majella Kenny, Paul Sales and Lesley Chrimes. I am glad to say that the two drug teams now have large numbers of staff, with the only 'downside' to that being that I cannot acknowledge them all here. In this edition I will have to restrict the 'name-checks' to those who have given me material that they have worked on which I have used in the book: Simon Brown (amphetamine prescribing), Rod Dutch (buprenorphine detoxification), Ciaran Fahy (drug polices – although I know he would not want to be linked with all the opinions I have put forward in the book!) and Gemma Malpas, medical student (alcohol use by opioid treatment patients). I am indebted to my excellent consultant colleague in Sheffield, Dr Olawale Lagundoye, who is Clinical Director of our service and has definitely been flexible in his requirements of me at the height of the book deadline! Regarding this, I have been grateful indeed to Richard Marley and Katie James, the editors at Cambridge University Press, for the combination they have shown of patience and encouragement.

The most fulfilling part of our work in drug misuse treatment is helping the patients overcome their problems and improve their lives, even though I would be the first to acknowledge that this does not always run smoothly! Some reviews of the first edition of the book pointed to the mixed and intermediate outcomes which are illustrated in many of the contained case histories, and looking back I am sure that this was deliberate, to reflect the realities of treatment on the ground. Most of the histories have been retained and others are new, and I have been careful to make them composite rather than exposing the identity of single individuals.

Mark Parry and I hope that the cases, the descriptions of the range of treatments which can be used and the discussions of wider aspects are of interest and assistance to those working in drug services or determining overall policies, and we are grateful for your interest in the book.

Introduction: community treatment in context

In providing clinical treatment for drug misuse we play one part in addressing a problem which is among the most serious facing modern society. The use of illicit drugs has escalated hugely in recent years in many countries across the world, with wider causes which are beyond our control as, indeed, are any overall solutions. Most of the trends which have led to such high rates of drug misuse show no signs of abating, and political arguments rage as to the relative merits of differing social policies and approaches to drug legislation. Within this, as clinicians we have a specific prime responsibility to treat individuals who present with identifiable drug problems, plus an additional implicit role in helping those affected by such use, and we must be able to fulfil these as successfully as possible as part of the much bigger picture. This requires an informed knowledge of all the approaches which can best help individuals to stop taking drugs or to reduce their usage in their various personal situations, and can limit the associated problems in homes, families and communities.

This book aims to help in that task by reviewing from a practical standpoint the treatments which are indicated across a broad range of clinical situations. In recent times the treatment scene internationally has been dominated by methadone, the so-called 'heroin substitute' which can enable users to avoid the various consequences of taking illicit drugs. The substitution approach is inherently controversial, in that it necessarily replaces one drug of addiction with another and has no real equivalent in the way we manage other dependencies, but it is undoubtedly here to stay, with strong evidence for general effectiveness in severely dependent individuals. With ever-broader usage, however, including in the attempts to stem the HIV epidemic, the problems and limitations of methadone have become increasingly apparent, and the alternatives which may be safer or less addictive, or offer other clinical advantages, are reviewed here. There is also a more general concern among workers in services that the emphasis on opioid maintenance treatment completely skews presentation rates so that, unless positive steps are taken, little attention is paid to users of non-opiate drugs such as cocaine, or to less dependent individuals. I have included a review of treatments for misuse of the wider range of drugs, while at the heart of the book is an account of the methods of helping users achieve detoxification from heroin and other opiates. Candidates for possible detoxification rather than methadone maintenance can only increase as heroin becomes widely available and more and more young people begin using it; services need to target such individuals, to offer treatment before addiction becomes established. The deployment of community services is described, and there are discussions of the important aspects of practical provision for various clinical groups. Our own services have a strong community psychiatric orientation, which includes the principle of working with primary care physicians wherever possible, and many of the treatments which are described in the book are also applicable in that setting.

The number one priority in writing the chapters which follow has been to examine *realistically* the treatments we use in day-to-day practice, with reference to many of the problems which can occur in managing this often difficult population. In terms of an additional theoretical perspective, undoubtedly the social aspects of drug misuse are those which are particularly emphasized. As a clinician in this field it is impossible not to be struck by the social considerations at virtually every turn – in the associated problems of individuals, characteristic subcultural aspects in different types of usage, social origins of drug use, social consequences, and in the nature of many of the benefits of treatment. This dimension of the drug misuse phenomenon will be a recurring theme throughout the book, so that, for instance, the next chapter recognizes that the social effects of methadone treatment are as striking as any other kind, raising fundamental issues about the nature and purposes of this treatment approach.

This introductory chapter takes one step back from the treatment situation, to examine the social background against which drug misuse is often set, some of the aetiological factors, and the place which clinical treatment occupies in the wider scheme of things. It is by way of a fairly subjective and partly historical overview, before the treatment approaches are examined in greater detail, in various international contexts. In our own services we use inpatient or residential options only very rarely, and so they are summarized at the end of the chapter, with some additional consideration where relevant in later chapters.

Drug misuse as a social problem

The use of various substances has very different meanings in different cultures and countries (Westermeyer 1995). In addition, attitudes to drugs do not remain static, but change over time, as recently witnessed in relation to cannabis. In general, however, in blunt behavioural terms, it may be said that the taking of any drug which is currently illegal, whatever we may think of the legislature, represents a more 'deviant' behaviour than taking a drug which is legal, however harmful that drug may in fact be. In many countries, clinically significant illicit drug use often arises in the context of other broadly antisocial and marginalized activities, being associated in the same geographical areas and, to varying degrees, in the same individuals. Concentrations of drug misuse occur in environments with high levels of school truancy, gang activities and various types of crime, and a history of these may be found in those presenting for drug treatment. In such situations, even when a genetic theory of substance misuse is tempting, for instance if a parent has been a heavy drinker, lifestyle factors can seem just as important, with each generation using the available substances as part of a general behavioural and social pattern. Reviews of actual familial transmission in substance misuse are referred to below, while we can speculate that the social influences may be even stronger in those outside treatment, for whom drug use may be effectively a recreational activity.

In cities and towns particularly, the rates of drug use and other antisocial problems appear to increase steadily, with ever-younger individuals involved. The social causes are no doubt similar to those in the condition of personality disorder which have been carefully examined by Paris (1996a): these include family breakdown, parental psychopathology, weakening of the effect of authority systems and social disintegration in communities, in which there are reduced constraints on antisocial behaviour. With the demonstrations of increased prevalence of drug use, including school surveys, the activity can be said to have become more normative over the past few decades. In such circumstances the levels of associated problems and psychopathology among those who use drugs may be expected to be less, but this has not been convincingly demonstrated, and it can equally be claimed that in countries where there is widespread drug misuse, this is partly an indicator of generally extensive social problems (Kraus et al. 2003).

There is clearly a big difference between the occasional use of cannabis and dependence on 'hard' drugs in the various social aspects, including the context of usage and, especially, the social consequences. Much of the widespread recreational drug use may produce no discernible social problems, with the exception of the consequences of legal sanctions if caught. However, as usage progresses, and in a kind of gradient across the range of drugs, social consequences may include family and relationship problems, isolation from those except other drug users, reduced job prospects, debt, crime and adverse effects on child care (Jaudes et al. 1995, McMahon & Rounsaville 2002). The relationship with crime is not a straightforward one, and even acquisitive crime by drug users cannot simply be explained by funding expensive drug habits. Increasingly those involved in crime and antisocial behaviours will tend to use illicit drugs as a lifestyle feature, just as they tend to smoke. Whatever the connections, the criminal justice system can be a good place to engage drug users to offer advice and treatment, and arrest referral schemes have become commonplace.

With such strong social factors operating, many clinicians outside drug misuse treatment take some persuading that the condition significantly represents a clinical one at all, as opposed to a problem requiring social solutions. However, the general syndrome of dependence has strong psychological elements and, as we shall see, can be effectively addressed in drug counselling, provided an assertive enough clinical approach is adopted. Psychiatrists have a definite role because of the predominance of associated psychiatric problems, albeit usually the partly socially defined ones of conduct and personality disorders, and there is the whole area of medical management of complications. Most basically, drugs are substances with complex actions on the central nervous system, and the more that drug dependence progresses, the more clinical its treatment becomes. Within this, there is no doubt that social benefits are necessarily part of the aim of treatment, and the exploration of the unusual position of providing pharmacological treatments directly to achieve such outcomes begins in the next chapter.

Risk factors for drug misuse

As well as the very extensive work on aspects of neurobiology (Lingford-Hughes & Nutt 2003, Volkow & Li 2004) and genetics (Fowler et al. 2007, Ball 2008), social and psychiatric research have both made substantial contributions on the subject of the aetiology of substance misuse. An unfortunate aspect of the literature is that there is little connection between these disciplines, so that subjects such as unemployment or social disadvantage on the one hand, and personality or psychopathology on the other, tend to be discussed without much acknowledgement of areas of overlap. Table 1 indicates some of the risk factors for drug misuse, and the main contention here is that the personal and social factors are importantly interlinked.

Within the personal factors, clearly family disruption, trauma and physical or sexual abuse can all predispose to conduct disorder in adolescence and personality disorder in adulthood (Paris 1996b, Spataro et al. 2004). Links between such factors and subsequent substance misuse have been consistently found (Bartholomew & Rowan-Szal 2002, Poikolainen 2002), while the associations between established personality disorder and drug

Table 1 Related risk factors for drug misuse

Personal	Social
Disrupted family of origin	Deprivation
Childhood trauma	Poor environment
Abuse	Frequent adverse life events
Adolescent conduct disorder	Relationship problems
Educational difficulties	Unemployment
Antisocial personality disorder	Lack of social opportunities

misuse are among the strongest in the clinical literature (Seivewright & Daly 1997, Grant et al. 2004). In terms of interconnections, the range of background problems can produce difficulties in forming and sustaining relationships, and personality disorder is associated with high rates of ongoing adverse life events, which are usually seen as social factors (Heikkinen et al. 1997). Personal factors may also lead to unemployment, as may educational difficulties, which predispose to drug use partly through disengagement from the school system. Lone or unstable parenthood is associated with substance misuse in adolescent children (Ledoux et al. 2002), but such parents are at increased risk of both psychopathology and disadvantage in housing.

A short review of the demonstrated relationships between social deprivation and drug use was provided by Pearson (1996). He notes not only the correlations with unemployment, but also the 'local informal economies of crime and hustling which thrive in areas lacking opportunities for involvement in the formal economy'. As if the risk factors for drug misuse were not related enough, he also describes the melting pot effect of problem housing estates. 'Tenants largely comprise those who cannot obtain anywhere preferable, including the previously homeless, teenagers in their first accommodation, women escaping domestic violence, and the elderly poor. If drug misusers are also added, or arrive through squatting, drug use can spread rapidly in fertile ground.' This scenario, compounded by a lack of other social opportunities, is very familiar to those of us providing services in large cities.

The role of treatment

Given the complex nature of the phenomenon which comprises the various forms of drug misuse, what is the role of treatment, and who should receive it? Drug services certainly need to concentrate their efforts on providing treatments which are effective, and the later chapters are aimed at shedding light on that aspect. Even the concept of effectiveness is not straightforward, however, and in our multi-faceted subject we must avoid being trapped into too narrow a concept of 'evidence-based practice'. Giving methadone is a fundamentally different type of treatment to many others offered in drug misuse and, not surprisingly, has the strongest supporting evidence by far, but it is wrong to provide that to the virtual exclusion of other approaches which may be entirely suitable in many cases. Substitution therapy is hardly used at all in non-opiate misuse, including the very major current problem of cocaine misuse, but it would be completely wrong to avoid seeing such cases and attempting to use the techniques we do have.

The two simplest answers to the question of who to treat are: those who want to be treated, and/or those who have an established problem of definite dependence. (The management of medical and psychiatric complications can be seen as a separate issue, although there is much overlap in practice, as will be discussed.) Such selection has become somewhat diluted in recent years, following the involvement of drug users in the HIV epidemic, and then the increased emphasis on crime reduction, with consequent initiatives of injecting equipment provision, harm reduction advice for those who continue to use drugs, and generally more accessible treatment. Also, in terms of motivating factors, there are many probation-linked schemes for those who may not otherwise have sought treatment, but who comply as an alternative to custody. While the need for approaches like these is undeniable, the broadening of acceptance criteria poses a number of problems which should be acknowledged, and which with a colleague I examined in more detail in another practical review of treatments (Seivewright & Iqbal 2002).

First, the number of referrals can rapidly become unmanageable. Although it is impossible to know the true prevalence of drug misuse for any area, in a city of 600000 people such as our own, Sheffield, the number using opiates, cocaine or large amounts of amphetamines is probably more than 10000. Even the best-established treatment service would have problems coping with one-fifth of that number, and resources are simply never going to be available to cater for the full demand. Second, there may be a distinct lack of impact if treatment is offered uncritically to those in whom drug use is basically a symptom of multiple social problems, as discussed above. Although the presence of other problems is absolutely no bar to treatment, and indeed looking at drug use can be a 'way in' to offering consistent professional help with various general benefits, the role of drug treatment in such circumstances must not be overplayed. Third, with a wide variety of types of drug misuser presenting from different referral sources, prioritization can be extremely problematic, especially if some emphasis on what may be broadly termed motivation is to be retained.

In many ways it is useful to have drug services operating on two different levels. Basic facilities such as injecting equipment provision, information, advice on a drop-in basis and supportive counselling must be made widely available. There is then a need for *clinical* treatment services, to provide the range of specific behavioural interventions and pharmacological treatments for individuals with problems, with access maximized but some limitation inevitable. In community-based treatment services it is usually a guiding principle to offer some treatment to as many users as possible, and the operation in this way of our own services and of community drug teams in general is discussed further in Chapter 5.

The overall response to drug problems includes prevention, education, treatment and enforcement. To debate the appropriate relative contribution of these elements is beyond the scope of this brief discussion, but it is clear that all organizations involved with drug misuse largely fail to keep pace with the extensive rates of the problem, or to make significant impressions on the drugs scene in general (Adrian 2001, Reuter & Pollack 2006). Non-enforcement prevention initiatives have tended to drift towards 'secondary' prevention, basically a form of harm reduction, in effect accepting ongoing drug use. The effects of drugs education are largely unproven, but at the same time those who know at first hand the difficulty of managing established cases of drug misuse should accept that, if possible, prevention is better than attempted cure. Meanwhile the criminal justice systems in many countries simply do not have the capacity to deal with all the drug offenders, and sentencing is often light across the range of drugs. The changing role of enforcement was discussed by Hellawell (1995), who became the UK's first antidrugs coordinator ('drug czar'), while an important point which affects the balance between the various systems is that not all forms of drug misuse are equally amenable to treatment. As we shall see, nearly all the established specific clinical interventions are for opiate misuse, including the option of substitution, which has no real parallel in other drug problems. The more challenging nature of managing non-opiate misuse is often not appreciated by other agencies, and drug services need to advise others realistically about the potency of clinical approaches, in situations such as diversion from court.

Inpatient and residential treatment

Inpatient treatment

This may be used for detoxification from one or more drugs, management of medical and psychiatric complications, initiating substitution treatments in particularly problematic cases, or various forms of respite. Some services use admission for dose titration in all patients starting on methadone or buprenorphine, but this is rare. For detoxification it seems fairly clear that a specialist unit for drug misusers is usually a preferable setting to a general ward. Apart from the difficulties which drug misusers and general psychiatric patients may have in getting on with each other, staff need to be well versed in matters such as obtaining urine samples and restricting visitors and time off the unit, and in various complications which are characteristic in such admissions. There need to be treatment contracts of some kind, and on a specialized unit there can be a therapy programme designed for drug users, rather than attempts to fit in with more general options. At worst, some nonspecialized staff have little sympathy for the condition of drug misuse and withdrawal discomfort, which can produce an angry response from users. In the UK, inpatient drug programmes are usually pragmatically based, with keyworker sessions and some group work focusing on areas such as coping with withdrawal, anxiety management, relapse prevention and drug-free lifestyles. There may be input from Narcotics Anonymous, while some units, particularly in the private sector, are based exclusively on the 12-step approach (Lile 2003). This has the advantage of being a very assertive and unequivocal method but, in our populations, drug misusers tend to accept it less well than alcohol misusers; indeed, combining both groups can itself sometimes be problematic.

The question of whether detoxification treatment in a specialist unit is more successful than on a general psychiatric ward was tested in a randomized trial by Strang et al. (1997). The specialist unit appeared more acceptable, with almost a quarter of those who were randomized to the general ward failing to accept that allocation, and fewer subsequently presenting for admission there than at the unit. Completion rates were also higher in the specialist setting although, importantly, that group received methadone whereas patients on the general ward had clonidine only. During seven-month follow-up, significantly more patients from the specialist unit had remained drug-free than from the general ward. A separate and very large study interestingly found better outcomes in opiate addicts who had been admitted from methadone maintenance treatment rather than directly from heroin use, suggesting that some of the behavioural changes already made in going onto a programme had been beneficial (Backmund et al. 2001).

Some of the more interesting options in opiate withdrawal are those that achieve detoxification more quickly than a standard methadone reduction. These can include the precipitation of withdrawal by opiate antagonists and even detoxification under general anaesthesia, and the various methods of inpatient opiate detoxification are referred to in Chapter 3. The clonidine analogue lofexidine is commonly used in the UK, which we prescribe, combined with other medications, as one method of quick community detoxification from heroin (see Chapter 3). Buprenorphine is also increasingly used in both inpatient and community settings as the most direct alternative to methadone, and this newer treatment is closely examined in Chapter 2.

Residential rehabilitation

This is a lengthy treatment, with rehabilitation centres often taking clients for 6–12 months or more for residential treatment. Some use 12-step methods (Gossop et al. 2008), while some are run by religious organizations or according to a strong 'concept' theme. In Sheffield we have one of the Phoenix House centres which are established internationally, and local colleagues have studied characteristics of their cases (Keen et al. 2001). Often, residential centres are away from main centres of population and, indeed, addicts are usually advised to go to one in another area, to consolidate their break from their drug-using scene.

Some centres provide a short detoxification, or this may be done just before going in. Often this is requested as an inpatient, to facilitate the transfer, and many inpatient services therefore prioritize individuals who have a rehabilitation place waiting. The group and individual therapy in rehabilitation centres typically concentrates not only on personal issues, but on making fundamental lifestyle changes. Very assertive tactics may be brought to bear to counter the behaviours that are seen as characteristic, including deception and exploitation. The treatment is demanding, but is intended to be somewhat more curative than clinical approaches are generally considered to be. Selection is very important, as many users are unable to truly make a commitment to a long-term residential treatment of this nature. Phoenix House in Sheffield operates a family unit, where drug misusers who are parents can have their children staying with them, with parenting assessments undertaken.

Topic in brief – 1. Community or inpatient treatment?

- In large-scale services inevitably most patients will need to be treated in the community
- Reasons for inpatient stays include full detoxification, stabilization, and management of complications
- Often more severe cases are admitted for detoxification, but premature discharge very common
- Specialist addiction units appear preferable to inclusion in general psychiatric wards

---

General observations

Inpatient hospital treatment and residential rehabilitation are very different in character, and in average length of stay. It is very useful to have both available as options for selected cases, but clearly they cannot be used at all routinely, because of the sheer numbers of drug users presenting, and the strong preference which most have for being treated from home.

Some general observations may be made, which to varying extents apply to the two settings. The assessment of cases for possible admission to an inpatient or residential unit should preferably involve a member of staff from the unit, to enable the most accurate briefing about treatment conditions, expectations and rules. This is especially important since, as with alcohol cases, there is something of a received wisdom that inpatient detoxification is indicated for those individuals who have too many adverse prognostic features to be successful at detoxification as an outpatient, such as heavy usage, long history, multiple drugs, personality disorder and poor social situation. In practice, not only are such individuals also perhaps the least likely to complete detoxification successfully as an inpatient, but they are often especially unable to tolerate the constraints of a hospital setting. Discharges for self-medication or behavioural disturbances are common, and in general a high degree of proficiency is required in these settings, and in assessment procedures, to avoid what may be termed a 'severity paradox', in which success is positively unlikely in those who are particularly considered to require the approach.

Exactly what constitutes 'success' is contentious in any drug misuse treatment, but one point is brought into particularly sharp focus in relation to the inpatient and residential options. This is the question of success at detoxification – do we mean just that, or are we by implication taking into account whether an individual actually stays off drugs afterwards? The purist view is well stated by Wodak (1994):

[Detoxification] should be considered successful if safe and comfortable withdrawal has been achieved, whether or not this is followed by a permanent state of abstinence. The ultimate achievement of abstinence, if that should happen, should be regarded as a bonus...detoxification should therefore be regarded as very different from other forms of treatment, and possibly should not even be considered to be a form of treatment.

In a review of the effectiveness of detoxification, Mattick and Hall (1996) say something similar:

Many countries adopt services that seem to be based on the belief that detoxification can bring about lasting changes in drug use, despite evidence to the contrary. Detoxification is more appropriately regarded as a process that aims to achieve a safe and humane withdrawal from a drug of dependence. This is a worthwhile aim in itself.

While the clear separation of the elements of detoxification and subsequent relapse prevention is indeed an important clinical principle, the sheer imbalance between outcomes in maintenance and detoxifications can be striking, with O'Brien (2005) for instance bemoaning 'the effort that must be expended to achieve an opiate-free state, no matter how transient'. Undoubtedly many observers, including those who fund treatments, would expect that the labour- and cost-intensive residential options should have a more lasting impact, to be justified. To take extremes, the situation of someone relapsing into heroin use one week after a short course of medication as an outpatient is less unfortunate than someone relapsing one week after 18 months of intensive residential therapy and, in fairness, the long-term rehabilitation centres generally accept that higher 'obligation'. As clinicians we must use the treatment methods that appear appropriate in each case, but in our own services, as in many others, we acknowledge that we strongly favour community treatment, mainly on the grounds of patient preference, but also to maximize the number of individuals who can receive treatment from limited resources.

The strongest traditions of inpatient detoxification relate mainly to alcohol misuse, in which the withdrawal syndrome is inherently more dangerous than that from opiates, and the avoidance of withdrawal complications in standard treatment may be the prime consideration in selecting admission. (In drug misuse, as we shall see in subsequent chapters, indications for admission increasingly relate to new developments, such as rapid detoxification techniques, or severe clinical states produced by crack cocaine.) The drug misuse treatment scene is very different from that in alcohol in many ways, but most notably because of the acceptance of a substitution treatment approach in the form of methadone, buprenorphine or alternatives, and this produces another problem regarding inpatient and residential treatment. Again as will be discussed in detail, methadone maintenance in particular has been strongly encouraged on harm reduction grounds since the threat of HIV among drug misusers, and clinicians have become nervous of opiate users being in difficulties without such medication. When a methadone or buprenorphine patient is admitted for detoxification, it is therefore difficult to strike the right balance as to how readily the substitution drug should be made available to them again if they run into problems. If it is virtually guaranteed that they can have their medication back should they prove unable to cope with the detoxification, that can have a major demotivating effect, while if that safety net is not there, users who might be able to detoxify will be deterred, and so the integration of approaches merits attention (Broekaert & Vanderplasschen 2003). Of course, this difficulty also applies to community detoxifications from opioids, but in the case of costly inpatient treatment the implications of aborting a detoxification to re-establish maintenance are magnified.

The particular problems of inpatient care and long-term residential rehabilitation for drug misusers are best addressed by those with a substantial commitment to such treatment, including services with specialist inpatient units for this group (e.g. Buntwal et al. 2000). Such units can offer a range of detoxification techniques and variable periods in which rehabilitation needs are examined, with appropriate assessment procedures, inpatient programmes and aftercare. In recognizing that such treatment is for a small minority, the rest of the book will describe the components of a community-based approach to drug misuse treatment.

Treatments

Methadone: the main treatment for the main presenting drug problem

Introduction

Opiate dependence is the type of drug problem presenting most frequently to clinical drug services, for two very strong reasons: first, the individuals are overall the most ill, with their undoubted physical withdrawal symptoms and other complications, and secondly, there are medical treatments which are routinely applied. These are not just any medical treatments, but the potent force of a direct 'substitution' method is frequently used, with agonist medications prescribed which in theory can immediately relieve individuals of the need to use their drug such as heroin. Even if the opiate addicts were not severely unwell the availability of a substitute medication would no doubt skew relative presentation to services, and indeed this is given as the reason for concern that groups such as stimulant users have 'nothing to go to drug clinics for'. In many countries methadone has been the standard choice for substitution treatment, and in particular is reached for when it is thought that 'maintenance' will be required, i.e. that because of length of history and general problems there would seem little prospect of short-term detoxification being successful. It is again completely unsurprising that, as discussed throughout this chapter, the success rates for maintenance treatment in enabling individuals to stop or drastically reduce illicit drug use over substantial time periods are far superior to those for short-term withdrawal courses, and it is a matter of routine for methadone to produce reductions in other drug use, and in physical and psychological problems, injecting, social complications and crime (Hall et al. 1998, Marsch 1998, Appel et al. 2001, Luty 2003). It has been said that methadone maintenance is one of the most effective treatments for any kind of clinical condition, and the easy avoidance of acute social problems such as debt and acquisitive crime greatly contributes to such effectiveness measures when they are included.

The particular properties which have made methadone attractive for substitution treatment since the days of the early trials (Dole & Nyswander 1965) are indicated in Table 1.1.

In terms of bioavailability methadone is as satisfactory taken by mouth as by injection, and so the addict should be enabled to switch from the most hazardous form of heroin use, injecting, to taking a medication in oral mixture form. Methadone has an elimination half-life of around 24 hours, and so once-a-day dosing is generally advised, although as will be noted later there is great inter-individual variation in pharmacokinetics and sometimes twice-a-day is truly necessary. The subjective effects of methadone are stabilizing rather than euphoriant, and so in relative terms there is less temptation to over-use the medication than there probably is with morphine, diamorphine, etc. Finally it is very notable that after initial titration to an adequate dosage, the dose reached can remain satisfactory over very long periods, even if the mechanisms for this lack of increasing tolerance – which appears

Table 1.1 Desirable properties of methadone as a substitution (agonist) treatment in opiate dependence

As effective orally as parenterally
Long acting
Relatively non-euphoriant
Little need to increase dose over time

in addiction patients but less so in pain management – are poorly understood. Of course none of these matters is absolutely straightforward, so that for instance some patients seem to fare better on injectable than oral methadone, other individuals do appear to gain euphoria from excessive methadone and will take as much as they can at one time, and in actual clinical progress the effectiveness of methadone maintenance in stopping other drug use is often found to wane over time, and so such matters will be discussed. However, methadone mixture has become the 'gold standard' treatment across many parts of the world, and the general effectiveness has been uncontested since the early times when after several trials against placebo treatment these were considered no longer ethical to do (Newman & Whitehill 1979, Gunne & Gronbladh 1981).

Various studies have shown other medications to be broadly as satisfactory as methadone in improving physical and psychological wellbeing and reducing social problems in opiate addicts, but the extent of evidence is nowhere near as great. At one end of the spectrum of both euphoriant property and similarity to the drug of actual misuse there is pharmaceutical diamorphine, usually given in trials by injection, and, as will be discussed in Chapter 2, the advocates of that point out that only a minority of individuals can *fully* make the adjustment from street heroin to oral methadone and therefore stay off all drugs completely. Prescribing diamorphine definitely does not involve the behaviour changes that methadone treatment does, but seemingly a significant part of the effectiveness of maintenance with a substitution agent does not absolutely depend on the medication itself, with improvements also shown in studies of morphine (Eder et al. 2005), dihydrocodeine (Robertson et al. 2006) and even codeine (Krausz et al. 1998). The availability of the different medications varies across countries, but it has become very apparent in the last decade that the most similar approach to giving methadone, producing virtually equivalent results in many large-scale studies, is to prescribe sublingual buprenorphine (Mattick et al. 2004). This last will be the subject of a detailed examination in the next chapter, and has become the main alternative to methadone in the clinical situation of heroin or other opiate addiction. As a final initial observation, it has been very interesting to see the situation in France, where methadone had previously been very little used before buprenorphine was introduced as the first widely available substitution option (Guichard et al. 2003). The picture of greatly increased presentation of addicts to services and routinely achieved benefits in the kinds of indicators mentioned above was virtually a parallel of the introduction of methadone to other countries, again suggesting that it is basically the provision of a substitute that readily enables the broad benefits to occur. Of course chemically buprenorphine is a partial rather than a full opioid agonist, which leads to pros and cons in theory and practice as will be seen.

Having therefore acknowledged that the effectiveness of methadone probably relates partly rather than exclusively to the specific aspects of the medication itself, the large body of evidence will now be summarized as it pertains to this clinical treatment. The scale of the literature is vast, and while this book has its own emphasis in looking at practical aspects across a wide range of treatments in opiate and non-opiate misuse, readers are also directed to highly authoritative volumes on methadone (e.g. Ward et al. 1998a). In writing the first edition of this book I was keen to mention the main matters to do with methadone provision which seemed important in daily clinical practice and which allowed some consideration of the nature of this particular treatment, and I have kept to that principle.

The term 'methadone maintenance'

This term is used increasingly casually to refer to ongoing prescribing of methadone over any reasonably lengthy period. Usually a constant dose is implied, but sometimes slowly reducing courses are also described in this way. Strictly speaking, however, the term – especially methadone maintenance therapy or 'MMT' – refers to the highly structured programme approach which was originally devised for the delivery of methadone treatment in the USA, and is described next. This is not just a matter of semantics since, as will be seen, much of the systematic evidence for methadone's effectiveness relates to treatment as carried out in structured programmes, and the inference that any long-term prescribing amounts to approximately the same thing can lead to false assumptions about the process and the range of benefits.

Formal methadone maintenance programmes

It is well known that the concept of formalized methadone maintenance originates from the work of Dole and Nyswander (1965). The treatment was devised for established opiate addicts, and was based on the principle that, following the physiological changes which occurred through prolonged taking of opiates, the state of dependence represented a metabolic disorder which required corrective treatment indefinitely. The fundamental aspect of methadone treatment was seen to be not simply the relief of withdrawal symptoms and craving, but a 'narcotic blockade', whereby an individual on methadone would fail to experience the euphoriant effects of heroin if that were taken (Dole et al. 1966). This effect was considered to be due to cross-tolerance, and it was observed that methadone doses of at least 80 mg per day were necessary to achieve it. This relatively high dose was therefore prescribed on a long-term basis, with no intention that patients should attempt to reduce. The first clinical programmes were for recidivist addicts, with the related aims of reducing heroin use and crime.

A structured programme approach to the delivery of methadone treatment was con-sidered essential. Addicts were stabilized on high-dose methadone in a hospital ward, fol-lowing which they returned on a daily basis for supervised consumption of medication and urine testing. There was an initial comprehensive assessment of medical, psychiatric and social problems, with facilities to address these on an ongoing basis. Along with the provision of methadone, the addicts entered not only counselling, but also placements in education or employment. Relaxation of the daily attendance for methadone or urine screening was only for individuals deemed to be making excellent progress, although take-home doses for part of the day were also necessary for those who had difficulty spanning a 24-hour period with one dose. Programmes along these lines developed across the USA, with inevitably some differ-ences in provision emerging over the years. Ball and Ross (1991) undertook a clinical out-come study across six methadone programmes in the mid 1980s, and found a wide variation in programme elements and effectiveness. This research was considered to strongly support methadone treatment as it had been originally devised, with the most successful programmes characterized by high methadone doses, definite maintenance treatment rather than attempts at reduction, more intensive counselling and more medical services, as well as features indicating good relationships between staff and patients. Some replication was provided by Magura et al. (1999) in a larger sample of methadone clinics.

Other long-term methadone prescribing

Since methadone was introduced it has, in practice, been provided according to a very wide range of treatment models and policies. There are major differences in treatment internationally, which are mainly beyond the scope of this book but have been the subject of reviews (Bell et al. 2002, Solberg et al. 2002). Notwithstanding the strong evidence for the original approach, which is discussed further below, there has generally been a gradual departure from this, for various reasons which are interrelated. The overall trends in provision have been towards lower dosage, fewer additional interventions and less emphasis on outright maintenance treatment although, importantly, these do not necessarily apply together.

The dilution of the original approach within the USA has been partly due to financial and political considerations (Rosenbaum 1995), but many other influences have also affected services. As with other psychiatric conditions, ideologically there has been less acceptance of the medical model, and therefore, in the case of methadone, of the implicit need for life-long treatment. In the meantime, heroin has become more and more available, with a wider range of individuals presenting, who may require a long-term approach but not necessarily a universal high-dose policy. Also, elements such as special employment schemes have become much less common and, without these, routine daily attendance at a treatment centre has gradually been considered less acceptable, for those who are attempting to normalize their lifestyle in other ways.

Some of the changes which occurred in methadone treatment have come about as a result of the threat posed by the involvement of drug misusers in the HIV epidemic, really from the 1980s onwards. In the UK and other countries methadone was seen as an important vehicle for shifting heroin users away from the risks of injecting (e.g. Advisory Council on the Misuse of Drugs 1988), but it was recognized that the delivery of treatment needed to be substantially altered if it was to make an impact in public health terms. There was much emphasis on engagement in treatment, with methadone in effect attracting users into services so that other HIV-preventive work could be undertaken, and also on subsequent retention, with routine discharge from treatment for additional drug use considered inappropriate. This use of methadone for individuals who would in many cases not previously have qualified for definite maintenance produced more instances of ongoing low-dose treatment, and the retention aspect meant that there was more recognition of those who do not successfully modify their drug use to taking methadone alone. Rigid approaches were considered undesirable primarily because they may deter those individuals who pose some of the highest risks, while ideological considerations have been important in generally taking more account of individuals' views on their own treatment. In this way many 'low threshold' programmes grew up (e.g. Buning et al. 1990, Klingemann 1996, Langendam et al. 2000) with the overriding philosophies of easy access to treatment, harm reduction policies and individualized dosing.

Lower average doses of methadone have resulted not only from the drug being given to a broader population, but from heightened awareness of its side-effects and particular addictive potential. The addictiveness does not so much matter if treatment is conceived as being life-long, but relatively few patients in treatment fully wish this to be the case (Lenne et al. 2001). With abstinence often an ultimate aim, many individuals elect to be on the lowest comfortable dose of methadone with a view to gradually cutting down, and something of a hybrid between maintenance and detoxification emerged, variously referred to as 'maintenance to abstinence' (Department of Health 1991), 'abstinence-orientated maintenance' (Capelhorn 1994) or, latterly, simply 'reduction' (Gossop et al. 2002a, b). Apart from the aim to be off methadone, another very major factor in practice is reluctance of patients to take anything like a full 'blockading' dose of the medication, often preferring to take enough to 'hold' them (i.e. prevent them withdrawing) in the absence of much motivation – or necessity – to stop other drug use. This has become a dominant issue in modern treatment, and observations are made at various stages here and in Chapter 3.

Outcomes in time-limited methadone treatment have generally been found to be very poor in comparison with maintenance (McGlothin & Anglin 1981, Gossop et al. 2001, Magura & Rosenblum 2001), although the early influential studies were typically in established maintenance candidates who had treatment restricted, rather than individuals who chose to reduce as an option within a flexible policy. For our purposes this intermediate duration of treatment, which now applies just as much to buprenorphine, is classed as slow detoxification, and is discussed in the section on detoxification from the two medications.

Before examining other core elements including counselling and drug testing, some consideration will be given to the nature of methadone treatment itself, which again relates in part to the dosage issue.

The nature of methadone treatment

Specific treatment or heroin substitute?

A comparison between the medical model of methadone treatment and a model of methadone as a so-called heroin substitute is outlined in Table 1.2, and these concepts will now be considered.

The medical model of methadone treatment, as proposed by Dole & Nyswander (1965), was later reviewed by their co-worker Kreek (2000). The initial studies pre-dated the discovery of the opiate receptors and endogenous opioids, and methadone was selected largely on the basis of careful clinical observation in pain patients and in addicts. The clinical properties of long duration of action (24–36 hours) and effectiveness by mouth were considered highly advantageous, and in addicts the drug appeared to reduce craving and produce a 'narcotic blockade', referred to above. This approach to opiate addiction was widely taken up in the USA and elsewhere, and in this original concept methadone is seen as a straightforwardly medical treatment, resembling the use of insulin in diabetes or antihypertensives in high blood pressure. The early proponents stressed that in cases where dependence had become clearly established over a significant period, the treatment should be continued for as long as the patient wished and it was producing benefit, with Dole (1973) asserting that 'each withdrawal [from methadone maintenance] is an experiment with the life of a patient'. It has frequently been pointed out that the portrayal of methadone as a straightforward medical approach has been particularly necessary in the USA politically, where the concept of a substitute drug would fit uneasily with the strong emphasis on

Table 1.2 Medical model and substitution model of methadone treatment

	Medical model	Substitution model
Rationale	To correct metabolic disturbance caused by opiate dependence	To provide a reasonably satisfying drug effect
Mechanism	Reduces craving and blocks effects of other opiates	Reduces need to use other drugs
Explanation for improvements in health and well-being	Primary, due to methadone	Secondary, due to removal from street drug use
Dose	High	Minimum comfortable dose
Duration	Indefinite	Should be able to gradually withdraw

enforcement. The suggestion in this version of treatment is that it is the medication itself which produces the behavioural changes, but the substitution process is still implicated, if methadone acts to reduce craving for other opiates and to deter such usage through its blockade effect.

Alternatively, the substitution principle may be spelt out rather more directly, as it tends to be in European countries. (In the UK we are often considered to have a specific 'British system', but this is largely a separate matter relating to drug legislation and prescribing before the modern era of recreational drug misuse, although the concept does include our use of some injectable medications (Strang & Gossop 1994).) Broadly, the 'heroin substitute' view of methadone regards the provision of a guaranteed supply of legal pharmaceutical opioid as leading to a range of secondary benefits, as the activity of illicit drug-taking is reduced or (more rarely) stopped. Improvements in general health, mood and personality are therefore seen as indirect rather than direct effects of methadone, more related to avoiding the complications of other drug use. Indeed, methadone is truly a substitute for the preferred drug, heroin, and although the long-acting property and oral route are acknowledged as beneficial, in this view of methadone there is also more acceptance that individuals will actually vary greatly in their ability to adjust to methadone's much more limited subjective effects.

Although the concept of substitution is quite compatible with ongoing treatment, the issue of duration of methadone to some extent becomes tied in with treatment models. Thus, long-term maintenance has sometimes been referred to as 'medical maintenance', and short-term treatment as 'psychotherapeutic maintenance'. The implication of the latter term is that with additional therapy and support it ought to be possible for an addict to be 'weaned off' opiates using a reducing course of methadone. This presupposes that opiate tolerance gradually reduces during withdrawal, in an opposite process to the increase which occurs as dependence develops, whereas the medical model does not accept that the various neurobiological and neuroendocrine abnormalities in opiate dependence can in fact be reversed (Kreek 2000). This issue is far from clear-cut, as the medical model view is based substantially on the high relapse rates after detoxification, to which many kinds of factors may contribute, as well as on biological changes of uncertain clinical importance.

A classic example of different approaches

Such contrasting views of methadone treatment were tellingly encapsulated in a joint article several years ago in *Addiction* journal, which was followed by a series of commentaries (Ball & van de Wijngaart 1994, Wodak et al. 1994). On a visit during an international harm reduction conference, Dr Ball, who carried out some of the main formative work in the USA on beneficial elements of methadone maintenance programmes, and Dr Wijngaart, an expert on Dutch drug policy, had interviewed a client at the methadone clinic in Utrecht, The Netherlands. In a frank discussion with the programme director and other visitors, the client described his many previous attempts to come off drugs, and related that he had reduced his methadone to 12.5 mg per day. He was not hopeful of completing his methadone reduction, but said that he was 38 years old and he wanted to be changing his life and seeing more of his two children. Unfortunately, as well as his methadone, he was still taking a wide range of other drugs by injection, and he believed that many other clients in the programme did the same. The two authors gave their different views of this situation, with Dr Ball regretting that 'somewhat surprisingly, [the client] seems uninformed about the pharmacology of methadone maintenance and the need for long-term treatment'. Dr Wijngaart observed that the client was 'a typical Dutch methadone client', from a background of using many different kinds of drugs and probably quite unable to adhere to only methadone. Habitual drug users were entitled to 'seek detoxification to regain their health temporarily or because they really want to stop their drug dependence', but the main purpose of methadone was to keep a wide range of clients in contact so that other harm reduction measures could be deployed.

The issue of whether it is inadvisable to attempt to detoxify from maintenance treatment is a major and controversial one, and again some of the salient points are well illustrated in an article from the relatively early days, this time a study by Eklund et al. (1994). It was carried out in Sweden, within a USA-style methadone policy where there was no requirement to detoxify from established maintenance treatment. However, 59 out of 600 patients had voluntarily done so, and their outcomes were investigated, at an average follow-up of seven years. The high number of seven had died, and two were untraceable. Of the remaining 50, 25 had successfully withdrawn from methadone, 19 at the first attempt. Of those, however, five had current substance misuse problems, mainly with alcohol. Twenty-five had resumed methadone maintenance and had usually achieved good stability, but quality-of-life measures were generally better in those who had succeeded in withdrawing from methadone. In this group who were very long-term drug users, therefore, it appeared that attempting to withdraw from methadone maintenance was indeed risky, with a tendency to substitute with other substances, but that if it could be achieved, it resulted in a better quality of life. Similar issues have been considered in more recent work from the same treatment institute (Hiltunen & Eklund 2002).

In this book methadone and other candidate medications are referred to as substitution treatments, and that broad concept is employed rather than the purely medical model. It is considered that one of the main reasons why long-term methadone treatment produces such good results is that it does not require those who have risk factors for ongoing drug misuse, such as personality disorder or an adverse social situation, to be completely without the effects of a mood-altering drug, albeit that those effects are intentionally limited in the case of methadone. Further, it is relatively easy to avoid other substances of misuse, given that a drug is provided, and so there are consequent reductions in many other indices of drug use such as injecting or HIV-risk behaviours. As indicated at the start of the chapter methadone can be seen as being partly nonspecific in its impact on drug-taking patterns, but is undoubtedly the most proven medication in attempts to convert individuals from street drug use to the clinically more desirable effects of a prescribed regime. It is clear that many opiate misusers cannot make this transition completely, and there need to be alternatives such as those identified in Chapter 2.

The following case history includes several features which are reasonably characteristic of progress in treatment with methadone, as delivered in a community setting.

Case history

Chris was a 24-year-old man who was single, but with a child from a previous relationship. He had an eight-year history of drug misuse, including cannabis, ecstasy, LSD and amphetamines, with heroin misuse for the past three years. He had initially smoked heroin, but progressed to injecting as he became more dependent, and at the time of referral was using 1–1.5 g per day. He had tried stopping several times himself, but had been unable to tolerate the withdrawal symptoms. He had had one methadone course from his general practitioner, but complained that this had reduced 'too quick', with heroin use restarting after the early stages.

It was agreed that Chris needed methadone treatment on a more prolonged basis. He was started on 40 mg per day, but two increases were required to go to 70 mg per day, on which he claimed to be entirely comfortable. Dispensing was at his local neighbourhood pharmacy, with consumption supervised except at weekends. He indicated that he did not want to be on methadone very long term, as he did not really see it as a solution, and believed it to be 'worse to get off than heroin'. There was no pressure from us to reduce quickly, and it was felt that an initial stabilizing period on the same dose was required.

At the first few appointments Chris's progress seemed excellent, with improvements in mood and general health. He was very pleased, and was wearing the new clothes he had been able to buy with money which he said would have previously gone on drugs. While continuing at the same dose, however, his urine drug screens still showed heroin products and, on one occasion, amphetamine, in addition to methadone. He told us his heroin use had dramatically declined, so that while he used to raise money illegally to buy heroin every day, he would now only have it if it was offered when somebody came round to his house. To his counsellor he admitted that although the methadone enabled him to avoid feeling ill, and he did not really crave heroin, there was something missing with the effect of methadone and he could not resist having drugs on an occasional basis as a 'treat'. He retained a desire to change his lifestyle so that he was not involved in the drug scene, and he was sceptical of the idea that an increase in methadone would help him stop his other drug use.

It was agreed that Chris's situation had greatly improved on methadone treatment, but he was advised that we would wish to see his urine become free of nonprescribed drugs. Chris felt that such a requirement would actually help him in his own efforts to avoid other usage. Three out of four urine samples since have shown only methadone, and while one indicated heroin use, he emphasized that this was an isolated occasion and that he managed to smoke the drug rather than inject it. Overall, the reduction in Chris's drug use and criminal behaviour has been evident enough for his ex-girlfriend to allow him to have contact again with his young son. So far he has agreed to remain on the same dose of methadone and, given the gains and the previous difficulties, this is considered appropriate.

Individual treatment or public health policy?

The issue in considering this dimension is not so much whether benefits to individual health or public health accrue with methadone treatment, as clearly both do, and both are important in different ways. Partly the difficulty is whether, if we have one eye on the public health agenda of reducing HIV transmission from drug misusers, and other wider agendas such as crime reduction, we can still apply the treatment that is best at any time for each individual. Since awareness of the risks of that particular infectious complication was heightened, followed by increasing recognition of hepatitis C and also schemes aimed at safer communities, opiate misusers have in effect been 'cushioned' by the use of methadone treatment. They are already unlike other types of drug misusers in being prescribed a closely related drug and, depending on treatment policies, in not being required to work towards abstinence; now methadone is also relied upon for engagement purposes, and to protect against relapses which might increase risk behaviours.

In relation to individuals and treatment populations, methadone has long been shown not only to reduce other drug use and injecting, but specifically to reduce HIV-risk behaviours (Capelhorn & Ross 1995, Marsch 1998, Sullivan et al. 2005), and sero-conversion rates (Metzer et al. 1993, Gibson et al. 1999). Because of these impressive aspects, and the benefits in the other areas referred to above, access to methadone treatment is generally encouraged, and in a low-threshold programme relatively few demands may be made. Criteria for receiving methadone are often not rigorous and, once in treatment, if it broadly appears that the harm-reduction aims are being met, there is a tendency for prescribing to 'drift' into the long term in individuals who are not necessarily definite maintenance candidates. This situation is compounded by the fact that public health-oriented treatment means maximum number of methadone patients, shorter appointments, less attention to individual drug-using situations, and less associated counselling to consider alternative management possibilities.

Even in undoubted long-term treatment, there is an uneasy mix between individualized treatment and the wider health and social aspects, as Raistrick (1997) has pointed out in a thoughtful article on the subject. Although he acknowledges that 'prescribing methadone as a public health or social policy measure is not necessarily incompatible with prescribing for individual treatment', he envisages a situation where different purchasers of health care might have different desired outcomes, which would in turn influence the nature of substitution treatment. A criminal justice system purchaser might fund some places with the express aim of reducing the harm caused by criminal activity, and so to maximize that outcome prescribing would probably be high dose, long duration and include the possibility of injectable drugs or diamorphine if they were more effective for individuals in that regard. Furthermore, if an individual was failing on treatment there would be a tendency to go 'up the tariff' or, at the very least, retain them in the programme. By contrast, a patient on an individual treatment 'ticket' could face discharge from the programme for similar lack of progress, if the goal was more to encourage progressive reduction of dependency. The apt observation is made that 'in the real world prescribing doctors are pragmatists, and the circle is squared behind the closed door of the consulting room' (Raistrick 1997), but increasingly 'a transparency of objectives' is required in our understanding of the various purposes of methadone treatment. The irony is pointed out that methadone is often paid for solely by health services, whereas the benefits extend widely into other areas, and it is rightly suggested that the criminal justice system and social services should also shoulder the financial burden, even if differential objectives would mean some adjustments in treatment methods.

Of the various possible roles of methadone treatment, the public health role which was so strongly emphasized in the era of the HIV threat required reassessment in the light of high prevalence rates of hepatitis C among injecting drug users (Wodak 1997, Hope et al. 2002). Although there have been many demonstrations of benefits of methadone maintenance in relation to indicators of HIV risk, the hepatitis C rates suggest transmission of this agent still occurred through the same time period, and this is seemingly much more transmissible than HIV through blood (although less so through sexual contact). Different kinds of injecting equipment sharing are implicated, and it appears that some of the behaviour changes advised to reduce HIV risk are not sufficient to avoid hepatitis C (Jauffret-Roustide et al. 2006, Muga et al. 2006), even with the provision of maintenance substitution treatments (Crofts et al. 1997).

Effectiveness of methadone

Comprehensive reviews of the effectiveness of methadone have been provided by several authors (Bertschy 1995, Marsch 1998, Mattick et al. 2002). Here, we will examine the subject enough to gauge the overall importance of methadone within services, and to make some links with the discussions of the nature of the treatment and its actual provision. The reviews make it clear, as we also have at various stages in the book, that the majority of studies demonstrating methadone's effectiveness are of ongoing maintenance therapy. The evidence generally becomes weaker as duration of treatment shortens through to detoxification treatments, and also to a certain extent as there is departure from the original model of formal methadone maintenance programmes.

Randomized controlled trials date mainly from the early years, as not only is it difficult to obtain consent from large numbers of dependent individuals to either receive or not receive obviously useful substitution treatment, but studies against placebo were soon deemed unethical. Of course as other substitute medications have appeared there is a new generation of randomized controlled trials of methadone against these, mainly buprenorphine, but these will be considered in the sections in Chapter 2 on each opioid candidate drug. Regarding the earlier trials, another fundamental aspect was that methadone needed to be investigated in rather atypical situations where treatment was not otherwise available, so that those randomized to no treatment would not receive the drug elsewhere. The first was by Dole et al. (1969) in recidivist opiate addicts who were due for release from prison. Entry criteria included at least a four-year history of opiate addiction and at least one previous unsuccessful rehabilitation attempt. Twelve individuals started methadone treatment, with 16 randomized to no treatment, and at 12 months the findings were overwhelmingly in favour of methadone maintenance. Indeed, all of the control sample had returned to daily heroin use and prison, while none of the methadone patients was using heroin daily and only three had been imprisoned. A larger study in a broader population was carried out in Hong Kong, where methadone treatment was not in other ways available (Newman & Whitehill 1979). The same entry criteria were used, with evidence of daily opiate use, and 100 male addicts were included. All subjects were stabilized in hospital on 60 mg of methadone per day, and were randomly assigned either to be withdrawn from methadone under double-blind conditions and then receive placebo maintenance, or to receive methadone maintenance, both groups also having additional counselling treatments. Methadone maintenance dose was determined by the patients and averaged 97 mg per day, and those who had more than six urine tests positive for heroin during the follow-up, or who missed six daily doses, were discharged from the programme. At 32 weeks only 5 of the 50 placebo subjects were still in treatment, as against 38 of the 50 methadone subjects, the pattern continuing to produce figures of 1 and 28 respectively at three years. A significantly greater proportion of the placebo group than the methadone group had been discharged for heroin use, but three deaths had all been in the methadone group.

A study in Sweden used similar entry criteria (Gunne & Gronbladh 1981), but added a period of intensive inpatient vocational rehabilitation to the methadone maintenance programme, and employed a sequential design. Once again, at follow-up after two years almost none of the control group had ceased drug use or made other satisfactory progress, while in the treatment group there were high levels of cessation of other drugs and gaining employment or further education. A further randomized controlled study by Yancovitz et al. (1991) is interesting in that it tested the effects of 'interim' methadone treatment, involving limited other services, in those awaiting treatment in comprehensive methadone programmes. Treatment subjects received high-dose oral methadone by daily dispensing, but no counselling or structured social rehabilitation. A total of 301 heroin addicts were recruited, and in the period of interim treatment the proportion of subjects receiving methadone who were shown by urinalysis to be using heroin declined from 63% to 29%, with no corresponding decrease in the control sample. There was, however, no change in cocaine use in either group.

The Treatment Outcome Prospective Study (Hubbard et al. 1984, 1989) included over 11 000 drug misusers who had applied for treatment programmes in the USA over a three-year period. The treatment approaches were grouped into methadone maintenance, residential therapeutic communities, and outpatient drug-free counselling, and there was an extensive series of follow-up interviews, some on selected subgroups of clients. The outcome measures in the study were illicit drug use, criminal activity, employment, depression and suicide, and statistical techniques were used to control for various confounding factors such as educational level and extent of previous treatment. This study forms some of the basis for the often-quoted view that results of treatment are generally better the longer that individuals stay in the treatment, as that applied to various outcomes in this research. Retention rates were significantly better in methadone maintenance than the other modalities, and regular heroin use and crime in that group both dropped from high levels to less than 10% of individuals, 1–3 months into treatment. A major analysis of the influence of retention on treatment outcomes has been provided by Farre et al. (2002), while Zhang et al. (2003) found a straightforward correlation between treatment duration and avoidance of drug use in the methadone patients among a cohort study of 62 drug treatment centres in the USA. Once again retention was itself more beneficial in methadone maintenance rather than other treatment modalities.

Higher methadone dosages have consistently been found in studies to be associated with lower levels of heroin use, improved retention in treatment, and to a lesser extent other treatment benefits over low dose (e.g. Ball & Ross 1991, Maxwell & Shinderman 2002, Mattick et al. 2004). Various definitions for high dosage have been used, with analyses of results therefore using different cut-off doses, but typically the distinction between high and low lies somewhere between 60 and 100 mg per day, with the relevant Cochrane review (Mattick et al. 2004) finding that overall the better outcomes were for more than 60 mg.

Suppression of heroin self-administration in opioid-dependent volunteers has been found to be greater at doses over 100 mg (Donny et al. 2005), and this relates to the 'three-level' effects of methadone, the implications of which we often have to contend with in our discussions with patients. Basically low doses of methadone will suppress opiate withdrawal symptoms in dependent individuals, and this is what a lot of patients mean when they say that their dose (which may be considered too low by us) 'holds' them. In medium to high levels of methadone there is less craving for opiates, and then at the highest doses there will be full narcotic blockade (Donny et al. 2002), but as already indicated the users themselves may not wish to take such dosages.

A number of studies add context in different ways to this broad-brush finding. For instance, some early contradictory results (Seow et al. 1980) suggested that benefits of high dosage are not necessarily demonstrable where that is reserved for individuals who have failed on low dose, since they may to some extent represent a more difficult group who are prone anyway to additional drug use. Hartel et al. (1995) found that heroin use was generally greater in those who were maintained on less than 70 mg of methadone per day, but the patients who used cocaine were more likely than others to use heroin at all methadone dosage levels. The importance of inter-individual differences in pharmacokinetics of methadone, with for instance greatly varying levels of relevant enzyme activity, has been examined in detailed studies (Rostami-Hodjegan et al. 1999, Eap et al. 2002, Leavitt et al. 2000), while Gerra et al. (2003) found methadone dosage important in better treatment outcomes, but so also were daily administration, good quality of interpersonal relationships and stable employment.

The following box indicates some main points for clinicians. With the strongest evidence favouring high-dose treatment, there would seem to be no justification for imposing an arbitrary and sub-optimal top limit on the amount of methadone given out, which I have seen in services. Because of the risk of diversion, however, in practice we can be much more comfortable prescribing higher doses if consumption of the drug is to be supervised, or some other undoubtedly secure arrangement is in place. I have already mentioned the situation which is common but often unexpected by observers in clinics, of patients wishing to be on lower doses of methadone than we would prefer for them. I would add that this is in services which routinely have supervised consumption of methadone, whereas if a lot of the methadone is 'take-home' there can be far more requests for large 'doses', sometimes for diversion to other people. In recent times more information has emerged on the possible cardiac side-effects of methadone in high dosage, and depending on developments this may yet have a major impact on discussions of optimal dosing, alongside the effectiveness evidence. This is considered shortly in the section on safety issues.

Topic in brief – 2. Methadone dosage

- Studies consistently show better abstinence from other drugs, especially opiates, on higher-dose methadone (e.g. > 60 mg per day)
- Patients often unwilling to have such dosages, for reasons including aim of ultimately coming off, previous experience of severe withdrawals, and lack of motivation to avoid combined usage
- In a climate of involving patients in decision-making, clinicians often reluctant to 'tell them they don't understand the pharmacology of their treatment'
- Arbitrary limits on dosage inappropriate

Table 1.3 Main areas of benefit in methadone treatment

Reduced opiate misuse
Reduced crime and imprisonment
Reduced HIV-risk behaviours (injecting)
Improved quality of life
Reduced death rate
Improved physical and psychological health
Reduced non-opiate misuse
College, employment
Reduced HIV-risk behaviours (sexual)

In the reviews cited in this chapter there is often some breakdown of findings into those relating to heroin use, criminality, HIV-risk behaviours, social rehabilitation and non-opiate abuse. We have noted that crime was one of the earliest indicators in methadone treatment, while the wider range of outcomes is formalized in drug misuse rating instruments such as the Opiate Treatment Index (Darke et al. 1992a). The main areas in which methadone treatment has been found to be of substantial benefit are indicated in Table 1.3.

The list gives the approximate order in which effects have been demonstrated in systematic studies, according to reviews and a prominent meta-analysis (Marsch 1998). There is clearly a very substantial social component to beneficial treatment outcomes, with quality of life, for instance, including family and personal relationships, social stability, finances and other aspects of social functioning. These are commonly among the main areas of improvement seen in clinical practice, behind the most direct effects of reduced opiate misuse and drug-related crime. The demonstration within studies of methadone patients gaining employment has generally decreased over time (e.g. Kott et al. 2001), probably due to fewer special schemes and the more usual provision of sickness benefits, with some differences found between countries. Reduction in use of non-opiate drugs by individuals on methadone is undoubtedly very variable, but generally – and unsurprisingly – less striking than the impact on heroin use. The data on mortality partly relies on comparisons with out-of-treatment drug misusers, including those refused treatment or discharged, who may differ in important ways from those who are retained; this subject is considered below. More limited is the evidence of an impact of methadone on HIV-risk sexual behaviours, as opposed to injecting practices (Stark et al. 1996, Gowing et al. 2006). This discrepancy, found in many studies, is again predictable, but needs to be acknowledged in view of the emphasis on methadone as an HIV-preventive measure. Also, there appear to be subgroups of drug misusers who are less likely than others to adopt even the safe injecting practices, such as those with antisocial personality disorder, other psychiatric problems, benzodiazepine abuse or various characteristic patterns of drug-using with peers (Darke 1998).

In Table 1.3 I have included the areas of physical and psychological health, which often do not feature in reviews. Methadone has significant adverse effects, as discussed below, and by no means do all patients report subjective improvements in health on the drug, as opposed to when taking street heroin or other opiates. However, if methadone treatment is adhered to, there is normalization of various circadian rhythms and endocrine effects including menstruation (Schmittner et al. 2005), and sometimes improved immunological function, although findings on this are mixed (Quang-Cantagrel et al. 2001). In addition, the various complications of injecting and of erratically using street drugs can be avoided. Improvements in psychological functioning on methadone, such as reduced anxiety, depression and other mood disturbances, have been consistently reported (Musselman & Kell 1995, Calsyn et al. 2000).

Associated counselling

Counselling is one of the main aspects of process which has been examined in studies from the early days of methadone treatment, and more recently. In general, once again, the most positive evidence is in favour of a systematic and comprehensive approach. McLellan et al. (1993) randomly assigned 92 methadone patients to three groups which differed in levels of psychosocial services, with the actual methadone treatment remaining the same. Some 69% of subjects who received virtually only the methadone prescription continued to use other opiates or cocaine, with lower levels in groups who received additional counselling (41%), or counselling plus on-site medical and psychiatric services, workshops on employment skills and family therapy (19%). There is other evidence supporting the addition of a wide range of forms of counselling to methadone maintenance, including motivational interviewing (Saunders et al. 1995), a therapeutic community-oriented day programme (De Leon et al. 1997), couples therapy involving partners (Fals-Stewart et al. 2001), and a tailored twelve-step programme, Methadone Anonymous (Gilman et al. 2001). The very specific form of behaviour therapy which is often called 'contingency management', involving material rewards for abstinence from other drugs, has been used with methadone patients (Preston et al. 2000), but much less so than in cocaine abuse, which differs in having no clearly effective pharmacological treatment (see Chapter 4). The low acceptability of formal psychotherapy in drug misusers has been recognized (Seivewright & Daly 1997), and was strikingly illustrated in a controlled trial of short-term interpersonal psychotherapy by Rounsaville et al. (1983). Only 5% of eligible patients agreed to participate in that trial, with around half of subjects completing the study treatment. Better results were shown in a study where the therapy was cognitive-behavioural in nature rather than dynamic (McLellan et al. 1986).

An early study which demonstrated that intensive treatment is not necessary for all methadone patients was by Senay et al. (1993). In a controlled comparison, some individuals who had progressed very well in methadone treatment were switched from a conventional intensive regime to a system of having medical and counselling appointments only monthly, with other relaxations in programme elements. Not only was stability maintained, as demonstrated by a range of outcome measures and urine testing, but the new approach was so much preferred that it was considered unethical to return those users to the more demanding regime. The authors observed that, for well stabilized patients:

the time spent in travelling to a clinic two or three times a week and then waiting in lines for methadone and/or for counselling…creates problems in getting or holding a job and significantly limits their ability to relate to their family. In addition, they are exposed constantly to non-recovering patients and experience this as additionally burdensome, as these are the very people they are trying to avoid.

Following the evolution of methadone treatment internationally, as summarized earlier in the chapter, in many clinics medical and counselling appointments are at about that monthly frequency, with general drug counselling mainly on an individual basis. In our experience it is preferable to have the two kinds of appointments as separate, with the drug counsellor – or as we say 'keyworker', with the term 'caseworker' being similar – spending some of his or her time discussing the methadone treatment, but also looking at wider personal and lifestyle aspects. Typical material for the sessions includes treatment dose adjustments (in conjunction with the doctors), tactics in cutting down or stopping various types of drug usage, dealing with trigger situations and 'cues', and liaison with other agencies involved, and this kind of keyworking is discussed further in Chapter 5. In a large treatment service not all patients can have drug counselling input, but we find it especially important at times of significant change, such as moving from maintenance to a planned detoxification attempt. A situation that can be tiresome in practice is when a patient on established maintenance fails to attend for counselling sessions they have requested, but then contacts urgently wanting a 'friendly face' to assist in some specific (and possibly manipulative) prescription-related request, but even these contacts can sometimes be used to advantage!

From studies, an interesting finding by Saxon et al. (1996) was that although the receipt of a standard amount of counselling benefitted patients rather than just having methadone alone, a particularly enhanced level did not provide added benefits, although by contrast more sessions were seemingly preferable in an investigation by Fiorentine and Anglin (1996).

Practical management

Increasingly, some of the observations which follow will apply to treatment with the alternatives to methadone, especially the widely used buprenorphine. Also there are related comments throughout this book, which is intended to have a generally practical orientation, while the applicability of policies will vary across different units and countries depending on guidelines, facilities, funding, etc. Nevertheless it is hoped that discussion of some of the most important issues which arise in day-to-day practice is useful at this stage. To provide some orientation about our own services, approximately a third of all patients are on definitely long-term methadone, with its usage based on broad general guidance (American Psychiatric Association 2006, Department of Health 2007): such patients have established physical dependence on opiates (usually heroin), at least two years of opiate use, previous unsuccessful experience of detoxification treatment or clearly severe history if no such prior treatment, and are preferably aged 18 years or over, although exceptions are necessary to this. Usually methadone mixture is used, in dosages of 40–120 mg per day, with dispensing at community pharmacies. We emphasize that methadone should replace heroin and other drug use rather than be additional to it, and encouragement, counselling and monitoring are provided with that aim. To some extent the requirements on patients depend on the nature and extent of their prescribed medication, which principle is discussed elsewhere at various points, and outright discharge from treatment for additional drug use is rare.

Treatment contracts

The nature of methadone treatment, and the common complications which often occur in respect of appointments and unplanned presentations, make some kind of contract between patient and clinic desirable. In health services the standard of information given to users about basic matters such as opening hours, appointment systems and prescriptions has improved greatly in recent years, while inclusion of the aspect of abusive behaviours which will not be tolerated, or notices to that effect, are increasingly standard just as they are in railway stations, driving test centres or other public service premises. Beyond these general aspects it used to be common for patients to sign a written contract about their treatment, often with some undertaking to avoid nonprescribed drugs and an acceptance of the sanctions which would occur if they were unsuccessful. Of course the latter aspect is rare now, but a document which explains the expectations which user and worker can have in the process of treatment can still be useful. These may be uniform, or else very specific, perhaps at stages of an individual's treatment where a particular change is under way.

Drug testing

Principle

It can rightly be stated that several studies find good correlations between self-reports of drug use and test detection results, although of course relatively high agreement would be expected if subjects are actually informed that a study of that type is taking place (Ward et al. 1998b). Some people feel this questions the need for testing, while the other type of criticism is that with the 'window' period of detection of drugs in urine being so short, additional drug use in programmes is hugely under-recorded (Goldstein & Brown 2003). In our own services we feel that attempting to run drug clinics without urine (or other) drug testing is like trying to do a diabetic clinic without measures of blood sugar, or one for hypertension without blood pressures. Whatever cuts are required in budgets for the services we do not reduce testing, and indeed it is seen as a matter of absolute routine, with a urine sample being standard for each patient before each medical appointment. Because this is the 'same for everybody' we have remarkably few arguments about sampling, as opposed to when I first arrived in Sheffield and sampling was occasional, and often protested against, as in ' well I'm one of those that says if I've had anything', as if other patients would readily admit to being the type to keep it quiet. A sample is simply the preliminary to any planned appointment, with the other analogy we use for trainees being that it is just like reading the wall chart of letters before going in to see the eye doctor! As the other main consideration it is felt that since we give out controlled drugs it is definitely not unreasonable to know what else is being taken, and in this way it generally seems as if a right kind of balance is struck.

Methods

The most commonly used method is urine sampling, with a standard range of techniques for detecting the different substances (Moeller et al. 2008). It is important that clinicians in training know that heroin itself does not appear in the urine, being quickly metabolized to 6-monoacetyl-morphine and morphine, and also that in most laboratories the detection period for drugs is about 2–4 days after usage, except for benzodiazepines and cannabis, where the period can be significantly longer. Some of the drugs have metabolites which are routinely detected, and probably many people in practice have occasionally seen methadone appearing but no methadone metabolite (and perhaps a green colour to the urine!), indicating that a little of the medication has been tipped into a supposedly valuable drug-free sample.

In the routine large-scale opioid maintenance clinics we do not always do instant testing, with the sample going instead for full laboratory analysis. Of course if some decision about treatment actually depends on that day's result an instant test can be used, and these are now of high reliability. The giving of urine can be observed, but the sometimes low acceptability of that has led to mouth-swab testing becoming popular as there are no doubts about authenticity (Bennett et al. 2003). The fluid which is collected is oral mucosal transudate (i.e. not saliva), by osmosis, and the detection period for drugs is about the same as urine, or somewhat shorter.

By far the most comprehensive information comes from hair sampling (Tassiopoulos et al. 2004), preferably from the head, which has a reliable rate of hair growth of 0.75–1.5 cm per month. Most drugs remain detectable in hair for as long as it is growing, and so a properly taken sample according to the test manufacturer's instructions gives an indication of which drugs have been used in particular periods (e.g. 3-cm/3-month sections). This is generally too expensive to use in routine clinical practice, but increasingly it is done when much depends on complete abstinence from drugs, e.g. when children may be returned to the care of drug-misusing parents, or an addicted healthcare professional might return to work.

Topic in brief – 3. Drug testing

- Usually provides the main objective evidence of clinical progress
- Urine is the most common method, but mouth swabs ensure authenticity and hair testing much longer-term information
- If opportunities are sought to cut treatment costs, this is not a suitable area!
- Testing of opioid substitution patients should be for a range of drugs, because of the tendency to switch from heroin to other substances

---

Safety issues

There is not space here to identify all the risks in methadone treatment and the policies which are necessary to limit these, and additional reviews should be studied on the extremely important subject of methadone deaths (Webster 2005, and see below, including on the possible role of heart conduction defects). Certainly as a starting point anyone involved with methadone should be acutely aware that a single dose is readily fatal for a non-tolerant individual – of the order of 10 mg or less for a small child, and around 40–50 mg for an adult (Luty et al. 2005). At a time when an addict in a clinic might be prescribed 100 mg or more per day, as is so widely advocated, and a degree of 'flexibility' is introduced with reduced pick-ups perhaps because of temporary work, it is common to see amounts of methadone being dispensed which could kill about a dozen people (or far more children). There was a well-publicized case in our own city of a child fatally ingesting their mother's methadone while she was smoking heroin in the next room, and at the time of writing there has just been national coverage of another similar case. Few situations portray drug treatment in a worse light, and the cases illustrate breaches of the frequent advice for methadone consumption to be supervised in patients who are still additionally using heroin or other drugs, because of the likelihood otherwise of erratic combined usage.

Thankfully such advice is inherent in the UK's latest national guidelines (Department of Health 2007), but so is an extremely strong emphasis on retaining patients in treatment even if combined usage is occurring. With such guidelines being the first documents reached for by solicitors in malpractice cases many clinicians feel virtually unable to terminate episodes of prescribing no matter how poor the progress or erratic the contact, in the face of inclusions such as the following:

A decision to temporarily or permanently exclude a patient from a drug treatment service or provide coerced detoxification should not be taken lightly. Such a course of action can put the patient at an increased risk of overdose death, contracting a blood-borne virus or offending. It may also increase the level of risk to children and vulnerable adults in the home. If at all possible, patients excluded from a service should be offered treatment at another local service or setting in a way that minimizes risks and maximizes opportunities for patients to be retained in treatment.

(Department of Health 2007)

In this advice there is not even any exclusion regarding individuals who have simply been abusing the treatment service, for instance (as happened to us recently) by storing huge quantities of take-home methadone in their house as part of their dealing activities.

At the very least in the present climate we must all face the prospect of managing combinations of drug use much of the time, knowing as well that the risks from methadone are increased by concomitant use of drugs such as benzodiazepines, cocaine and alcohol (Worm et al. 1993, Coffin et al. 2003, Man et al. 2004). Of course this all falls under the established arguments for 'harm reduction' (van den Berg et al. 2007), but with re-starts of methadone in patients who have not picked up for a few days either because of crises or general disorganization being virtually a daily occurrence in services, and only about a quarter of individuals staying off other drugs on maintenance (Flynn et al. 2003), the distinction between accessible treatment and disorder can be rather fine. One visitor to local services told me that he thought methadone treatment in the UK was rather like 'an inoculation programme in a deprived country', and far from fundamentally disagreeing I find myself often quoting this when advising trainees of the nature of the work! For some, the most telling statistics when discussing how accessible and 'low-threshold' to make services are the low levels of HIV in addicts in those countries that have adopted such flexible principles (Farrell et al. 2005, van den Berg et al. 2007); the ethos was most strongly emphasized when involvement of drug users in a potential epidemic of that emerged, and so the recommendations to avoid very restrictive programmes seem to have been correct. Even for the doctors who are fearful of continuing giving methadone in the presence of additional drug use, reassurance has so far been provided by not only the data referred to earlier showing (virtually linear) benefits from retention in treatment, but also an overall *reduction* in mortality in patients on methadone maintenance (van Ameijden et al. 1999, Brugal et al. 2005, Fugelstad et al. 2007).

In the previous edition of this book I discussed in detail the repeated 'swinging of the pendulum' when the problems of over-restrictive and then over-flexible policies respectively accumulate, and already in the UK we are seeing the abstinence agenda become quite strong again, sometimes indeed through service user representation. With the surrounding arguments raging it is important to know the actual facts such as the mechanisms by which methadone is fatal, as discussed by Wolff (2002) and Corkery et al. (2004). As already suggested, the movement for high-dose flexible methadone treatment to be provided in as many settings as possible might be pulled up in its tracks by the worrying emerging evidence for heart conduction defects produced by the medication (Justo et al. 2006). It is known that the QT interval in an electrocardiogram can be prolonged by methadone, particularly in very high dosage, at its most serious risking ventricular tachycardia, and it is indeed possible that some of the deaths in the methadone-taking population which have been assumed to relate to respiratory depression or combination with other drugs could have involved this complication, undetected. There are signs that practitioners are concerned that ECG monitoring will be seen as required practice, with something of a consensus emerging that a cut-off point for this could be 100 mg a day of methadone. The complication appears to be commoner in females, which tends to apply with most drugs that do have the side-effect of QT prolongation. Also in terms of safety considerations there must be awareness of naloxone, which reverses fatal opioid effects and which in some schemes is provided to users for when they are present at an overdose (Strang et al. 2006).

Finally of these main observations, one area which is directly under the control of individual prescribing doctors is titration onto methadone, and it is well-established that caution needs to be the watchword (Payte 2003). The Department of Health guidelines (2007) point out that the toxicity of methadone at initiation is delayed, and relates to the half-life, which is very variable and affected by extraneous factors, and furthermore that different responses between individuals cannot be reliably predicted. The subject has been carefully much examined, and the principle of 'start low and go slow' (i.e. in increasing) is surely correct. A contrary view is sometimes expressed that patients might reject such doses and disengage, thus posing more risks, but in practice this seems very rare if suitable explanations are given, and if immediate cessation of other drug use before an adequate dose is established is not expected.

As with any other medication prescribing there must be awareness of drug interactions, with important ones for methadone relating to antivirals, psychotropics, anticonvulsants and antibiotics.

Topic in brief – 4. Balancing security and accessibility

- Very restrictive methadone programmes with routine discharge for additional drug use have become largely unapproved
- If there is additional drug use the opioid should preferably be given under a secure arrangement, mainly supervised consumption
- Prescribers often worried about the risk of increasing methadone dose in combined usage, but overall high-dose methadone reduces both such use and mortality
- Sometimes compromises necessary in policies and consumption arrangements, e.g. to avoid disengagement of the most generally risky cases

---

Additional medication

As far as possible, methadone treatment should mean just that, not methadone plus other medications of potential misuse. The theoretical footing for this is that the majority of the positive evidence for effectiveness relates to methadone alone, although we noted earlier that the main studies did not include individuals who were significant users of non-opiate drugs.

Those of us in countries where high-dose methadone maintenance is not unequivocally promoted must concede that we are likely to have more difficulties with additional psychoactive medication use in treatment. The most problematic drugs are the benzodiazepines, which are sometimes taken to enhance the effect of methadone (see Chapters 3 and 4), that combination therefore being more 'necessary' at lower dose. In our clinics we generally aim to eliminate benzodiazepine usage, but in those who wish to avoid a high methadone dosage and are capable of abstaining from illicit drug use on the combination, or who fail to respond to psychological treatment of associated anxiety problems, prescribing of benzodiazepines is sometimes accommodated. Given the nature of drug misuse clinics, any prescribing of benzodiazepines to some individuals will result in others seeking to obtain them without clinical need, and so, as to some extent with the opioid drugs, a general policy is important to establish as well as individualized treatment regimes (see Chapter 2 for discussion of prescribing of benzodiazepines and other sedatives).

Indications for other psychotropic medication such as antidepressants and anti-psychotics are basically the same as in other patients, but practical aspects are important. The drugs may not be able to be included in the same prescribing and dispensing arrangements as methadone, but a drug misuse clinic which is psychiatrically based will often wish to take these on rather than the primary care physician, to more easily ensure regular control. The risks of inappropriate usage also apply to items such as analgesics or nutrition supplements (which are sold to body-builders), but there may need to be some sharing of prescribing for financial or other reasons. In cases of dual diagnosis with severe mental illness it is preferable for a general psychiatry service to be involved with aspects such as depot antipsychotic medication, but this may fall to the drug misuse service if there is better attendance at the methadone clinic.

Adverse effects

The most serious direct risks of methadone treatment are from overdosage, which are considered above and are heightened by combined use with other drugs. The next, at least potentially, is a disordered heart rhythm termed polymorphic ventricular tachycardia or 'torsades de pointes', which can occur with higher-dose treatment and again if other drugs are also prescribed. The finding is probably more common in females and HIV-positive patients, and particular care is required in individuals with other heart problems, but, at the present time at least, the risk of progression to major arrhythmia or fatality is not considered sufficient to require routine cardiovascular screening of individuals going on methadone (Justo et al. 2006). Otherwise, methadone appears to be remarkably safe for long-term use, causing no recognizable functional deficits or somatic damage (Kreek 1978, Ward et al. 1998a). Novick et al. (1993) compared the health status of 110 patients who had been in methadone maintenance treatment for at least ten years with a control group of long-term heroin addicts, and found no clustering of unusual medical complications or abnormal laboratory results in the methadone group. Patients often need reassuring on this point, as many have the idea that methadone causes damage to kidneys, liver or other systems.

There are a range of more 'minor' adverse effects, however, which are often not mentioned in formal reviews of methadone treatment but which are discussed more in practical handbooks. In clinical practice these can be very problematic, variously leading to distress for individuals, limitations in compliance and requests for alternative treatments, and the most troublesome such effects are listed in Table 1.4.

The full list of adverse effects of methadone resembles those of morphine, as they are common to the opiate group. These include nausea, vomiting, dizziness, mental clouding, dysphoria, euphoria, constipation, increased biliary tract pressure, respiratory depression, drying of respiratory secretions, sweating, lymphocytosis and increased plasma concentrations of prolactin, albumin and globulins. Tolerance may develop more slowly to methadone than to morphine with respect to the depressant and sedative effects, which is linked to some of the dangers in the early stages of treatment (see above) and problems of sedation clinically. Effects that are possibly more associated with methadone than other

Table 1.4 Common adverse effects of methadone

Constipation
Sweating
Weight gain
Dental problems
Nausea
Amenorrhoea
Depression/lethargy
Reduced sexual desire

opiates include lethargy, feelings of heaviness in arms and legs, itching and other skin problems. Also, cognitive impairments in terms of attention, memory and problem-solving have been demonstrated in methadone maintenance patients compared to non-heroin-using controls (Darke et al. 2000), which may partly be explained by associated factors such as higher rates of alcohol dependence and head injury, but are of concern when improved self-care and normalized personal functioning are aims of treatment (Klein 1997). Mintzer and Stitzer (2002) found a wide range of impaired cognitive functions in methadone patients compared to controls, having excluded individuals who tested positive for alcohol or benzodiazepines.

In the course of clinical treatment with methadone, certain situations relating to adverse effects are characteristic. Nausea is a general opiate effect, but complaints most frequently relate to the methadone mixture. This preparation does have a syrupy consistency, but the problem for clinicians is that the alternatives – sugar-free mixture or methadone tablets – are both more injectable, and therefore requests or implied requirements for these are often manipulative. So are requests for the antiemetic cyclizine tablets, which are crushed and injected by drug misusers along with injected methadone. As indicated in Chapter 4, thankfully these particular claims have become less common now that guidelines are much more discouraging of any use of methadone tablets.

The other adverse effects commonly complained of in relation to methadone mixture in particular are weight gain and dental problems. Weight gain can be striking, as illustrated below, but, contrary to frequent suggestions, cannot be accounted for by the calorie content of the mixture, as a 50 mg dose is apparently equivalent in this way to eating about two biscuits. There is therefore no indication to switch to an alternative form of methadone on these grounds, and it appears that the reasonably strong association between obesity and methadone treatment (Novick et al. 1993) may be due to a direct effect of the drug. Other relevant factors are that heroin addicts in treatment generally gain weight as they stop injecting and encountering minor infections and also develop a more sedentary lifestyle, although arguably in the case of methadone the latter may be associated with the lethargy that many patients complain of. In practice, we find that very excessive weight gain virtually only occurs in patients who are on high-dose methadone (over about 80 mg per day) and are mainly avoiding street drugs. In lesser degrees, weight gain is a reasonable general indicator of compliance with treatment, although some individuals do not experience it, presumably due to constitutional factors.

Regarding dental decay, methadone mixture is a culprit, because of the reduction in saliva, an effect of the acid on tooth enamel, and syrup constituents leading to the growth of plaque (Bigwood & Coehelho 1990). Once again, however, the situation is not straight-forward, as there may be high consumption of snack foods, poor oral hygiene, infrequent attendance for dental check-ups or treatment, and masking of toothache by opiates. If alternatives to methadone mixture are considered unsuitable, patients can be advised to drink methadone through a straw or clean their teeth after taking it.

The side effects listed in Table 1.4 are generally those which cause most distress to individuals in treatment. Unfortunately, there are few useful treatments, so that in con-stipation the best approach is a high fibre diet and high (non-alcoholic) fluid intake. Sweating seems only partly accounted for by the histamine release, with other mechan-isms produced by methadone likely, and there may be some benefit from treatment with biperiden or the antihistamine desloratidine (Al-Adwani & Basu 2004) or, as we have found, propantheline bromide. Amenorrhoea is due to high circulating prolactin levels and has the effect that pregnancy is often only recognized relatively late. Some couples falsely believe that pregnancy is not possible on opiates or methadone, and need advising on this point. There may be reduced sexual desire, which ties in with complaints of lethargy and depressed mood, although sexual dysfunctions may also be present (Brown et al. 2005).

In their generally favourable study, Novick et al. (1993) found an increased rate of diabetes mellitus in methadone maintenance patients, which they ascribed to the same causes as the obesity finding, namely high calorie intake and sedentary lifestyle.

Case history

Stefan is a 26-year-old patient in our methadone clinic. He had been dependent on heroin for five years before presenting to the service, and clearly required substitution treatment on a probable long-term basis. His heroin usage was substantial and although, in the early stages of treatment, we attempted to manage him on 80 mg of methadone mixture per day, he required increases to 120 mg in the ensuing months. He felt that this dose was satis-factory, in that he was free of any withdrawal symptoms and felt mentally well, with no strong desire to use heroin. Occasionally, urine samples would show that he had used the drug, but this proved to be mainly on the days he received his benefit money, and he responded well to specific advice from his keyworker about avoiding this. For the past year his only additional drug use has been of benzodiazepines, on an irregular basis.

Stefan has always had a big build, previously being an active sportsman. However, whereas his usual weight had been around 210 lb, this has increased on methadone to 330 lb. This is a source of distress to him and more particularly to his wife, who finds his appearance embarrassing, especially as he has also developed excessive sweating. When questioned, Stefan states that he has little energy and rarely undertakes any physical activity, although this is compounded by the fact that he is reluctant to leave the house. He claims not to eat excessively in general, but he has a craving for sweet foods and has some chocolate every day.

Despite the problems, Stefan cannot contemplate being without methadone, or even reducing his dosage, which he unsuccessfully attempted at one stage. He feels that his life has improved in all other ways since giving up heroin, and he is fearful of risking a return to the drug-misusing lifestyle. He accepts the physical side effects, and in reality has little motivation to attempt weight reduction, for instance at a gym or a class. In view of his general satisfaction and his strong dependence on methadone, alternative approaches are not considered realistic at present.

Other forms of methadone, including injectable

Liquids

The form of methadone usually used in addiction practice is the mixture, 1 mg in 1 ml. In the UK addicts often mistakenly refer to this as linctus, but the linctus is a different strength preparation, 2 mg in 5 ml. The linctus can be useful when individuals are at very low methadone dose, since measurement is easier, but alternatively the mixture can be diluted. As noted above, a sugar-free version of the mixture can be used in those concerned about dental problems, calorie intake or nausea, although the grounds are not strong, and the sugar-free form has previously been easier to abuse by injection. More concentrated liquids (e.g. 10 mg in 1 ml) are particularly useful for automatic dispensing machines.

Tablets

The 5 mg tablets tend to prove unduly popular with patients if they are made available. Sometimes the reasons are genuine, such as carrying tablets to work rather than a bottle of liquid, but the tablets are also both more sellable and more injectable. They are a better proposition to sell as they can be seen to be unadulterated (whereas mixture may have been diluted), and so with the risk of their being crushed and injected, and with no real benefit of tablets for services, their prescribing in the UK is increasingly discouraged. As regards complaints of inability to take the mixture because of nausea, a policy of offering methadone suppositories in those circumstances dramatically reduces such claims!

Steels et al. (1992) reported their experience of attempting a change in prescribing policy, from the use of methadone tablets to methadone mixture, in a large UK clinic. The change aroused extreme hostility, with a rise in threatening behaviour towards staff. Wider effects included increases in the number of pharmacy burglaries and in the street value of methadone tablets, and the change was ultimately unsuccessful, with over three-quarters of the patients receiving tablets again three months later. Vomiting was the most common claimed adverse effect of mixture, but this was confirmed in only two cases.

Injectable ampoules

In the general discussions of methadone, we have noted that one of the most advantageous clinical properties is that it can be taken orally. There are a proportion of patients, however, who manifestly cannot give up injecting, and in such cases the use of methadone ampoules may be considered at least preferable to injecting street drugs. The treatment therefore perpetuates the aspect of injecting, and so the clinician must be certain that advantages accrue from the treatment which outweigh this. The usual circumstance would be that evidence of complete absence of street drug use is required for injectable methadone to be continued. Almost inevitably, before this treatment is used, there will have been prolonged failure to progress on oral methadone, with harmful injected use of other drugs which has a prospect of being eliminated if the step-up is made to injectable treatment.

In a survey of community pharmacies in the UK, Strang et al. (1996) found that of 3593 methadone prescriptions 80% were for oral liquid, 11% for tablets and 9% for injectable ampoules. For a long time the prescribing of ampoules was simply a pragmatic approach for some seemingly intractable injectors, and was not subjected to controlled clinical trials. However, the feasibility of doing a randomized trial of supervised injectable versus oral methadone was demonstrated by Strang et al. (2000), with broadly similar benefits resulting in reduced illicit heroin use and other health and social measures. The injectable treatment was much more expensive, and probably for this reason and the current recommendation for supervised injecting (Department of Health 2007) the use of ampoules will simply not become anything like routine, even in special groups. Some of the most comprehensive treatment units in the UK do use injectables (e.g. Sell et al. 2001), but with increasingly restrictive guidelines the transition is more likely to be from ampoules to oral mixture, with some positive practical experience documented of this (Myton & Fletcher 2003).

In the rare cases when injectables are used instead of methadone mixture, in our view the treatment contract must be correspondingly stricter. The abstinence from street drugs mentioned above is virtually mandatory, the principle being that if an individual persists in using additional drugs, although they will not be discharged from treatment, they can do so on a routine mixture prescription, rather than on one which has several disadvantages from our point of view such as expense and the requirement for injection. There should be daily dispensing, even if supervision facilities are not available, whereas the pharmacy study by Strang et al. (1996) found that prescriptions for ampoules and tablets were actually less likely to be on a daily basis than those for mixture.

Ampoules come in various strengths, including 10 mg, 20 mg and 35 mg (all at 10 mg in 1 ml), and three 50 mg options, in 5 ml, 2 ml and 1 ml. The concentrated ampoules offer the benefit of less liquid for those who have difficulty in venous access, but the 50 mg in 1 ml in particular can cause troublesome stinging at the injection site. The ampoules are primarily intended for intramuscular injection, but in this indication it is accepted that drug misusers will use them intravenously where possible. Often peripheral veins cannot withstand this for long and the femoral vein will be used, for which services may give instruction.

The term 'needle fixation' is sometimes used by patients and others, but the existence of this beyond an ordinary 'route preference' for drugs by injection is probably rare. Sometimes users will describe toying around with needles and water to satisfy an urge, by way of backing up their claims to be on injectables, but the decision to prescribe should be based on sheer evidence of persistence of injecting over time, rather than on this particular and questionable phenomenon. In a review which summarizes the limited systematic data on the results of injectable methadone prescribing, Sell (2003) includes with approval some clinical criteria previously suggested by Sarfraz and Alcorn (1999): basically current opiate injecting, previous unsuccessful treatment with oral methadone even in high dosage, absence of severe mental health problems and significant use of additional drugs, no medical contra-indications to intravenous administration, and a demonstrated ability – despite lack of success in treatment – to cooperate with attendance and drug testing.

The most considered examination of needle fixation has been by Pates et al. (2005), who point out that it is not a single entity, and may have a range of background factors and different presentations. They include a definition, and also acknowledge that there is an alternative sceptical view, which could – I suggest – be summed up that 'needle fixation is what you say you've got if you're going to a service that sometimes gives out injectables, and you want some'. For what it is worth, having heard the term virtually every day from hopeful patients at the height of the methadone tablets/ampoules/cyclizine abuse

33

phenomenon, I have hardly encounted it in recent years since ampoules have been much less 'on the menu', but of course that does not mean it does not exist, and reading of the review is recommended.

Case history

Michael is a 30-year-old man who has been a patient in our methadone clinic for three years. He has a ten-year history of opiate use in all, but previous treatment had been elsewhere on a detoxification basis. At one time he had strongly wished to come off drugs completely and went into a residential rehabilitation centre, but although he completed the stay satisfactorily he relapsed into heroin use soon afterwards. It is now agreed between us that his metha-done treatment will need to continue long-term.

On an established dose of 70mg per day of methadone mixture Michael showed a good improvement, but it was clear he was not able to abstain completely from other drug use. He lives in an area where heroin and cocaine are both easily available, and these drugs regularly showed in his urine drug screens. He considered heroin his main problem, strongly desiring the effect of that drug by injection. He could avoid this for a while, but the desire would build up and at least once a week he would need to have a 'fix'. After he had done this he would feel exasperated that he had spent money on drugs, with this causing particular problems between him and his girlfriend. He was strongly encouraged and advised to adhere only to methadone, but he would not have been discharged on the grounds of other drug use, since there had previously been exceptional social decline between periods of treatment.

After much discussion it was decided that Michael could have 70mg of methadone in injectable form on one day per week, with methadone mixture on the other six days, with daily dispensing. On this combination it was required that all urine samples showed no other drugs, otherwise his treatment would revert to methadone mixture as previously. At first, appointments and urine sampling would be every two weeks, moving to monthly if there was good progress. Since this combination was instituted all Michael's urine tests have shown methadone only, and he is quite satisfied with this approach. He says that if he gets a strong desire to inject in the middle of the week, he knows that his injectable methadone is coming on Friday and this is enough to dissuade him from buying anything else. His girlfriend is equally impressed, and their relationship, and the wider ones with their families, have greatly improved. For the first time, however, he is beginning to have problems with his injection sites.

2

Treatments
More than methadone? The case for other substitute drugs

Introduction

For all the evidence in support of methadone, clinicians cannot fail to observe that not all dependent opiate misusers progress well on the treatment, even when it is made available over prolonged time scales and in high dose. There may be any number of reasons for this to do with individual circumstances and clinical situations, but the nature and properties of the drug are also important. One problematic group are those users who appear to find it impossible to adjust to the relatively noneuphoriant nature of methadone, desirable though that property is conventionally considered to be. They will continue to use other drugs, often in direct combination with methadone, to gain more euphoria and so, as well as all the important considerations of motivation which such behaviour raises, the adequacy of the substitute drug must be called into question. If a maintenance methadone user persistently combines their drug with for instance benzodiazepines, cocaine or alcohol, ostensibly to gain effects more like those of heroin, it can be argued that fewer problems would result if heroin were actually prescribed, rendering the other drug-taking behaviours and risks unnecessary.

Most interest in this way has indeed focused on diamorphine, but other opiates have also been used with a similar rationale, and the first part of this chapter examines the relevant arguments and the limited available evidence. The subject arouses strong emotions, with some authorities finding it incomprehensible that anyone could apparently ignore the evidence for effectiveness of methadone, which is unparalleled in drug misuse treatment, to consider alternatives on any frequent basis. Other clinicians pragmatically point out that, much though we may wish and encourage our patients to find methadone satisfactory, a substantial proportion of mainly long-term injectors manifestly cannot do so but retain some motivation for treatment, and that variations on the substitute prescribing theme can produce benefits in difficult cases.

Further situations in which methadone can seem an unsatisfactory substitution agent are towards the other end of the treatment spectrum. In uncomplicated maintenance treatment or for detoxification, the criticisms which are levelled at methadone relate not so much to the subjective effects, but to the aspects of addictiveness, abuse potential and toxicity. The issue of whether methadone is too addictive to be really suitable for detoxification is considered in detail in Chapter 3, and the controversial subject of methadone risks and deaths in Chapter 1. It is in the relatively milder cases of heroin dependence that buprenorphine treatment as an alternative to methadone has risen to great prominence in several countries, although, importantly, the condition definitely does not have to be mild for this medication to be used. Undoubtedly the introduction of buprenorphine is one of the biggest developments in drug-misuse treatment in recent years, and this option will be discussed in detail.

The development of physical dependence on opiates before treatment is one of the main reasons why substitute prescribing is considered necessary and appropriate in this group of users. Such an approach is mainly considered unsuitable in the case of other drug groups, but some clinicians argue that the principle can be applied with benefit to heavy amphetamine users. It is suggested that the distinction between physical and psychological dependence is scientifically unsatisfactory, that some heavy amphetamine users appear to closely resemble opiate users in their needs for treatment and harm-reduction measures, and that it is inequitable to deny this group an approach which has such an overwhelming effect on engagement in treatment. Some evidence from clinical experimentation with amphetamine prescribing is included in a general discussion here, although following largely negative results in a controlled trial the advisory climate in the UK is very much against this option (Department of Health 2007). The final section is a practical examination of the area of prescribing benzodiazepines to illicit drug users. Any such prescribing has inherent disadvantages and much potential for abuse, but in practice the situation arises extremely commonly, and a realistic appraisal of the issues and the limited appropriate indications is necessary.

Diamorphine

Prescribing diamorphine for heroin users has attracted the most attention outside our speciality as an alternative maintenance approach including, inevitably, much coverage in the media. Its proponents claim, among other arguments, that giving the noneuphoriant methadone to individuals who are used to heroin almost invites the additional use of other drugs, as a 'high' will often still be sought. It is argued that, having gone down the route of substitute prescribing, it is more logical to give the pharmaceutical preparation of the preferred drug, rather than a drug that only approximates to its effects. Some critics advocate this as a general policy, but current clinical use in areas where diamorphine is available for this purpose tends to be limited to particular patient groups with long-established addiction.

In the UK diamorphine has been used for many years as one of the treatments of opiate misuse, and currently occupies a minority position alongside much more extensive prescribing of methadone, and increasingly buprenorphine. These are given for the usual indication of dependent opiate misuse, and the vast majority of individuals in treatment will be encouraged to persist with one or other of methadone or buprenorphine even when there are difficulties. Diamorphine is used by some clinicians in a proportion of long-term injectors who have failed to progress on oral or even injectable opioid treatment, with very little prescribing of the drug outside this chronic, nearly always older group. The peripheral position of diamorphine within treatment around the time of this book's first edition was illustrated by a survey of the doctors who held the Home Office licence which specialists can apply for to prescribe the drug (Sell et al. 1997). Forty-three doctors in the UK had such a licence, with the majority of those prescribing diamorphine only doing so for between one and ten individuals. This presumably represented a small fraction of those clinicians' total clinical caseloads and, in a short section for comments, enthusiasm for this option appeared lukewarm. Ratings of global outcome of diamorphine prescribing were mainly split between 'good' and 'average', with some clinicians stating that they only held a licence because diamorphine had been initiated by colleagues, or that they used the drug solely for short-term treatment. There was evidence of some more extensive usage, however, with three doctors prescribing for between 33 and 100 individuals.

Prescriptions issued for diamorphine in the UK were analysed around the same time in a survey of drug-misuse prescriptions at community pharmacies (Strang & Sheridan 1997a). One in every four pharmacies were included, and 64 ongoing heroin prescriptions were identified, constituting less than 2% of opiate prescriptions to addicts. Three-quarters of the prescriptions were for ampoules, but there was some use of tablets, liquid and cigarettes. Mean dosage was over three times the dosage for methadone prescriptions, with dispensing usually on a daily basis. Metrebian et al. (1996) reviewed the subject from a clinical perspective, and provided some brief information from their own treatment service. In what the authors stated was the largest heroin-prescribing clinic in the UK, 50 individuals were receiving the drug in doses ranging from 30 to 300 mg per day, as determined by tolerance testing. Most prescribing was in the form of ampoules, and that review discusses injectable prescribing in general.

It is well known that the tradition of some diamorphine prescribing in the UK relates to the so-called 'British System' of drug control (Strang & Gossop 1994). Legislation in the 1920s effectively placed the control of heroin and other addictive drugs in the hands of doctors to protect their use as medical treatments, and the subsequent response to illicit drug misuse decades later included some maintenance treatment with the drug. An early clinical trial of injectable diamorphine against oral methadone was published by Hartnoll et al. (1980), in which many of the 96 injecting heroin addicts made an apparently satisfactory transition to methadone, although there were also some notably poor results in that group. The study was influential at the time in limiting enthusiasm for diamorphine, but some specialists feel that drug misuse is now very different in terms of subcultures and patterns of usage, and that re-evaluation is definitely indicated. In recent years the focus of research has shifted to mainland Europe, in particular the Netherlands and Switzerland, although there have been further studies in the UK (Metrebian et al. 2001), where an excellent review of the whole subject of heroin, ranging from history and usage through to international controls and treatment, has been provided by Carnwath and Smith (2002).

Much of the recent renewed interest was stimulated by a project investigating heroin prescribing for drug misusers in Switzerland. The background and early results of the project, which also included prescribing intravenous methadone and morphine, were described by Uchtenhagen et al. (1996). Methadone had been available in Switzerland since the late 1970s, but there was increasing public concern that drug misuse was becoming out of control, and it was apparent to the various authorities that large numbers of drug misusers had no interest in treatment as it currently stood. The project was planned very much along harm-reduction lines, the main aim being to generally reduce HIV transmission risks by attracting previously reluctant users into treatment, and retaining them, with more acceptable prescriptions. The emphasis on retention was such that prescriptions would not be stopped on the basis of additional drug use, unless patient safety was compromised. Injecting of the medications was on-site, which eliminated diversion, and there were apparently no major problems with general acceptance of the project, for instance in neighbourhoods. In clinical terms, heroin proved not surprisingly to be the most desirable of the three drugs, but was only satisfactory in injectable form. The project included a cigarette preparation for those who had never injected, but testing showed much of the heroin to be destroyed in the burning process. Over the initial six months the retention rate of the project was 82%, and there were reported reductions in other drug use, illegal activities and prostitution, and general improvements in social stability and physical and psychological health. The authors aptly concluded that

> providing pharmaceutical heroin in this project permits to attract addicts who fail in multiple other treatment approaches and give them a new opportunity to take courage and engage in a therapeutic and rehabilitation programme without being forced to abstain from their preferred substance. It is not assured yet, however, to what extent positive changes in health and social status will continue over longer periods of time, and to what extent a drug-free lifestyle can be reached by participants in a later stage.
>
> (Uchtenhagen et al. 1996)

In the Netherlands, two related randomized controlled trials found generally preferable outcomes for heroin prescribing as opposed to methadone alone, although notably some treatment was combined and some of the diamorphine was in smokeable rather than injectable preparations (van den Brink et al. 2003). A total of 549 addicts were included, and as in similar research in Switzerland it is claimed that the cost-effectiveness of the treatment is good (Dijkgraaf et al. 2005). Subsequent similar work has come from Germany, with an open-label multicentre randomized controlled trial of 1015 heroin addicts comparing injectable heroin prescribing or oral methadone over twelve months (Haasen et al. 2007). The heroin-prescribing group fared better overall in terms of the two main response criteria, improvement of physical and/or mental health and decrease in illicit drug use, with also higher retention, but there were more serious adverse effects in the heroin group, mostly complications of injecting.

It has been emphasized already that where the rare treatment of diamorphine is selected in practice it tends to be in injectable preparations for committed injecting users, and a theme in the trials of non-injectable preparations has been seemingly poor bioavailability and the need for much higher doses. In the UK and some other countries cigarette preparations have been tried (e.g. Marks et al. 1991), whereas there is also the option of making up powder for smoking on foil. This can involve mixing diamorphine with caffeine to lower the melting point (Klous et al. 2007), and at present this is an even more unusual option than prescribing injectable ampoules, probably as there is not even the necessity in non-injecting patients to try and reduce infective and other complications. It is possible that smokeable options could be useful for patients initially on injectable diamorphine to progress onto, but experience with this is very limited.

In all instances of prescribing diamorphine with the aim of patients avoiding street heroin there needs to be a laboratory marker substance detectable which can identify the latter, and it is increasingly common for laboratories to be able to do this. As with morphine much higher doses are required than with methadone, probably of the order of 400–600 mg per day for a patient who might be on 100–120 mg of methadone. In our clinics we have quite often found that patients will seek to increase their dose further, and in such circumstances it is useful to remind them that that is one of the reasons why diamorphine is not usually recommended as a treatment and methadone is, with methadone able to be at the same dosage for many years. The implication is that if there are too many claims that the dose is not 'holding', someone could easily rule themselves out of the diamorphine option, and with encouragement we have typically found that patients do indeed stabilize on an ongoing dose, even if initially they did not think that that would happen.

Case history

Amanda is a 33-year-old woman whose case we inherited after she had been prescribed diamorphine in controversial circumstances. She had previously been a patient of the methadone clinic but her progress had generally been unsatisfactory, and eventually she had obtained treatment with diamorphine from a doctor in private practice. Unfortunately the doctor did not have the licence required to prescribe the drug, but by the time the situation was discovered treatment had been established for several months. It was agreed that we would take her back into our service, where diamorphine could be prescribed on a legal footing while her case was being reassessed.

Reviewing her history, it appeared that she had used heroin by injection for five years before being first prescribed methadone. She was from a relatively isolated small town where the limited network of users had few links with treatment services. She used heroin with her then husband, and both were eventually referred to the clinic after he had been charged with supplying the drug. They separated soon afterwards, and while he remained in treatment for only a short period before leaving the area, Amanda has been receiving prescribed medication since that time.

She had never managed to stabilize on oral methadone, with virtually all urine samples showing morphine, benzodiazepines and/or amphetamine. She was prescribed benzodiazepines by her general practitioner, while she claimed to be unable to give up injecting heroin and she also drank alcohol quite heavily. Her methadone dose reached 120 mg per day, and for a short while before dropping out she was prescribed this in injectable form, but still she did not refrain from other drug use. She worked in a city department store, but her job was under threat because of frequent time off.

When she returned to the clinic following her period on diamorphine, she reported that she felt a prescription of that drug would be the answer to her difficulties. Because of her limited contacts with other users in treatment she did not actually grasp that this was a rare option, and she had been bemused by the problems of the legality of her prescription. She simply stated that she had 'never got on with methadone', claiming that it made her lethargic and depressed. She had particularly disliked the injectable form since it had damaged her veins more than street heroin ever had. On the grounds of obvious lack of progress with methadone it was agreed that we would prescribe injectable diamorphine, on a strict contract requiring absence of other drugs except benzodiazepines, which she now received on prescription in very small amounts. Her private prescription of diamorphine had in fact been inadequate, with a week's supply lasting only three days, and our own prescription was to be for 500 mg per day, daily dispensing, with the contract enforced by two-weekly urine testing.

Although the circumstances of Amanda receiving diamorphine treatment have been unusual, her progress is now exemplary. All urine samples indicate diamorphine use only, with her finding no need to take even small amounts of benzodiazepines. She drinks alcohol no more than about once a month, on nights out with her work colleagues. She takes no street drugs, and her social, financial and work situations have improved greatly. She injects three times a day, with no problems in still using her arm veins. The only difficulty she has with treatment is in envisaging any alternative approach, and it is very unlikely that methadone will be able to be useful in future.

Topic in brief – 5. Prescribing heroin to addicts

- Attracts controversy and media attention like few of our other interventions
- For clinical practice has largely been limited to 'last-resort' treatment of older long-term injectors in the UK
- The international research base is now wider and more satisfactory, with benefits demonstrated over methadone including less other drug use and greater acceptability
- Prescribed dosage needs to be high, and may be prohibitively so with non-injectable preparations because of poor bioavailability

---

Dipipanone (Diconal)

Diconal is a combination tablet of the opioid dipipanone and cyclizine, the effects of which are highly regarded by drug users experienced with pharmaceutical opioids. Following widespread misuse of Diconal tablets by injection, in the UK in 1984 it was added to those drugs for which a licence is required for prescribing to addicts. The survey of doctors by Sell et al. (1997) found only 13 doctors to have a current licence, with as many prescribers considering the general outcome of prescribing Diconal to be 'poor' as 'good', and since then the number of licensed doctors has not much changed (Metrebian et al. 2007). By any standards this would seem to have a very small place within the treatment spectrum, for use within specialist clinics for a minority of exceptional patients. An important feature of Diconal is that, like dextromoramide, it is much more euphoriant when injected than when taken orally, and so issuing tablets runs a high risk of misuse in this way.

Morphine

Because diamorphine is converted to morphine in the body, prescribing the two drugs may be considered broadly similar. However, the initial subjective effects of diamorphine are crucial, and morphine is often a less attractive proposition. In the early major trial of injectable drugs in Switzerland (Uchtenhagen et al. 1996), in which the morphine protocol was based on previous experience in the Netherlands, two of the morphine-prescribing groups were curtailed because of poor acceptability by participants. Of side-effects, histamine-like reactions on intravenous injection were most frequently reported.

However, some patients on methadone mixture claim that, of oral preparations, they feel better on morphine, usually in terms of energy and mood, and study evidence for this is accumulating. Of the adverse effects of methadone, weight gain, sweating and reduced libido may also be less problematic with morphine, and Fischer et al. (1996) reported high acceptability of morphine in this way, with the results of treatment being as good as with methadone. Similar findings were reported in a cross-over study by Mitchell et al. (2004), with morphine rating as superior to methadone in terms of weight loss, avoidance of side-effects, reduced craving for other drugs, and social functioning. Overall 78% of patients preferred the slow-release morphine, and 22% methadone.

It is this slow-release tablet form of morphine which has been most studied and used in practice, with one disadvantage of the liquid mixtures being that at standard strength very large amounts are required. As with diamorphine, it is important to be aware that much higher treatment doses are needed for morphine than methadone, with opioid equivalent tables often misleading in this respect (Carnwath & Merrill 2002). The dose relationship is non-linear, and so although 10 mg of methadone might be equivalent to 10 of diamorphine or morphine, there is great divergence at the higher levels, with the recent study quoted above finding the morphine requirement 4.6 times that for methadone. As with diamorphine, therefore, a common dosage in practice is 400–600 mg per day, with some related work to the clinical study finding once-daily dosing to be suitable (Mitchell et al. 2003).

Case history

Alan is a 32-year-old man with a 16-year history of opiate dependence. His formative years of drug-taking were spent in using not street heroin, but pharmaceutical opioids obtained from robberies of chemists' premises. In this way he would inject Diconal, dextromoramide, morphine and diamorphine ampoules, and a wide range of other drugs. He joked with us once that methadone was always the last to be used of any raided supplies because of its boring effects. He had had several prison sentences, and any contact with treatment services was often short-lived.

In the past five years Alan has made a great effort to move away from the criminal lifestyle and illicit drug-taking. He has been helped in this by his relationship with his girl-friend, who is from a very different background and supports them both with a full-time job. He has become a patient of our methadone clinic, and at his appointments they both emphasize their determination that he should have nothing to do with nonprescribed drug use. His lifestyle has become extremely restricted, but his main objective has been to avoid any activities which might lead to further legal problems or imprisonment.

It was very apparent that long-term substitution treatment would be needed, and he was initially maintained, after titration, on methadone mixture 70 mg per day. His requirement proved much more than this and, in increments, the dosage increased to 150 mg per day. He reported no major problems in stopping injecting, and superficially his progress appeared reasonable. He was no longer involved in crime, and his urine drug screens showed only benzodiazepines in addition to methadone. He was obtaining these from various contacts, and in due course it was decided that we instead should prescribe him small amounts of diazepam under controlled conditions.

Closer examination revealed a situation which was far from satisfactory. Apart from going to the chemist each day to collect his medication, Alan barely left the house, and his girlfriend reported that he had no interest in any activities. He was taciturn and depressed, had little energy and had become significantly overweight. He was avoiding other drugs but this appeared to be a daily battle, in which he was preoccupied with the lack of any discernible subjective effect from his methadone. It was not considered that he was under-medicated, partly as with or without benzodiazepines he usually appeared mildly sedated with slightly slurred speech. When pressed about his difficulties Alan gave the impression of being intensely frustrated, and we concluded that, even after years of trying, he had failed to adjust satisfactorily to methadone's limited effects.

It was felt that a trial period was indicated on an alternative oral substitute medication, namely morphine sulphate tablets, with Alan's girlfriend involved in overseeing his daily consumption because of his long history of abusing opioids by injection. Diazepam dosage was reduced as part of the agreement. After three months there has been a limited, but significant, improvement in Alan's condition overall. Although his weight has not decreased he has more energy and interest, so that he helps in doing some jobs around the house. He is apparently never intoxicated, but feels some satisfaction from the morphine effect after his doses, and there has been a general improvement in mood. No disadvantage is apparent in taking morphine, and this is to be continued.

Issues in prescribing euphoriant opioids

The above drugs have been discussed as possible substitute treatments which are more euphoriant than methadone. The evidence relating to their use is limited in comparison to that for methadone, and they seem likely for the time being to remain relatively peripheral possibilities compared to methadone and buprenorphine. The euphoriant properties have been identified as a rationale for treatment, and this has various implications both for the individuals concerned, and in terms of overall treatment within a clinic.

At an individual level, the issues are similar to those which arise in giving injectable methadone (see page 32). Unless routine usage is contemplated, there is no way around the fact that, in terms of general progress, users typically have to 'fail' at standard treatment to be considered for the options so far described. Also, a recurring theme in the discussions of alternative prescribing, whether it be additional benzodiazepines, injectables or euphoriant medications, is that the potential *disadvantages* are such that some major *advantage* needs to accrue if it is done, that usually being complete abstinence from street drugs as identified in a strict treatment agreement. The nature of the more euphoriant treatments makes it very important that security must be higher, including daily dispensing to avoid over-use; unfortunately the opposite can sometimes happen when a user, successful in securing an alternative treatment, persuades the doctor that he or she is experienced enough to manage less frequent collection. Prescribers should also acknowledge that giving injectables or diamorphine tends to be 'one-way traffic', with the policy difficult to retract once established. This may not matter in the context of outright maintenance treatment, and indeed the situation is not inevitable as some users do find the euphoriant prescription which they have been seeking too destabilizing once it is actually available, and wish to revert to methadone.

The prescribing of alternative opioids may cause wider problems within a clinic population. Once it is known that they are given in some cases, individuals who are basically making good progress in adjusting to methadone or buprenorphine may nevertheless be tempted to seek a more euphoriant medication. Even if they do not actually do this, there may be some unease if they see those who are making less progress 'rewarded' with alternative drugs. This, of course, begs the whole question of whether most patients are, or are not, seeking to make the various changes away from their previous types of drug use, but my own experience is that the availability of different prescriptions for some within a clinic does not lead to unmanageable and unwarranted levels of demand. In Sheffield, where we use the more euphoriant medications in some cases, although many patients experience common problems relating to the use of methadone the number of requests for these options is not high, especially now that buprenorphine is routinely available as an obvious alternative to methadone of often high acceptability.

Levo-alpha-acetylmethadol (LAAM)

There are various mentions in this second edition that forms of drug misuse common at the time of the first have passed over, and similarly some treatment options have become less available or advised. The major one affected in this way has been levo-alpha-acetylmethadol (LAAM), in which a few years ago there was increasing interest because it was a direct alternative to standard methadone which offered less frequent dosing, with likely advantages for patients on supervised consumption (Eissenberg et al. 1997). The duration of action of the drug is up to 72 hours, and so it was looking as if 3 days a week dosing could be routine, whereas although this has been done with buprenorphine it is more experimental, with daily dosing of the latter still standard. However, LAAM has been withdrawn from licence across many countries, with the European Union directive on this having immediate effect in 2001 (European Agency for the Evaluation of Medicinal Products 2001). The reason was the incidence of life-threatening cardiac disorders including those of ventricular rhythm such as torsade de pointes, so actually the complication which is being increasingly recognized with high-dose ordinary methadone (see Chapter 1). Some research with LAAM continues in a limited number of programmes (Jaffe 2007).

Buprenorphine

This has become the main alternative medication to methadone overall in recent years, following licensing in various countries, including the UK. This is the same buprenorphine drug that is used in analgesia as Temgesic, and indeed when the possibility of higher-dose buprenorphine for treatment of opiate dependence emerged, the authorities in the UK were particularly nervous of possible injected abuse of the tablets. This is because injected Temgesic was a major drug of abuse in the country for many years, with the combination of this and temazepam being a greater preference than heroin in many areas of Scotland and the north of England (Lavelle et al. 1991). Temgesic tablets are 0.2 and 0.4 mg, but for use in opiate dependence the therapeutic dose mostly lies between 4 and 24 mg (Ling et al. 1998, Petitjean et al. 2001), and so it has been gratifying to note that the widespread injected abuse which was feared has in general not occurred.

This partly of course is because as a direct alternative to methadone under similar policies, buprenorphine for opioid dependence (brand name Subutex) is often prescribed for supervised consumption in pharmacies, at least in the early stages until patients are free of other drug use. The treatment is best viewed as a substitution therapy, but as is well known the drug is actually a partial opioid agonist and partial antagonist, with this property having various clinical implications. The first is that treatment is rather more complicated than with methadone, since as well as the tablets being sublingual (because of poor oral bioavailability), more importantly the first dose has to be taken when the patient is in opiate withdrawal. If this is not the case and opiates are still circulating, the buprenorphine will actually precipitate an acute withdrawal state, which often has the effect of putting the patient off the medication for good. The mixed agonist–antagonist profile does, however, also confer advantages, as follows.

Rationale

The potential direct advantages which buprenorphine may have over methadone are indicated in Table 2.1.

Table 2.1. Possible advantages of buprenorphine over methadone as substitution treatment in opiate misuse

Safer overall
Quicker initiation onto effective dose
Less addictive
Less interaction with other euphoriant drugs
Sooner transfer to naltrexone after detoxification

The clearest advantage is that because of the antagonist effects there is a ceiling on the degree of respiratory depression which occurs, and so buprenorphine taken correctly is not dangerous in overdosage in this way (Walsh et al. 1994). If other drugs are also taken, however, there can be fatalities, as described with additional benzodiazepines or alcohol (Reynaud et al. 1998, Kintz 2001), and possibly death can occur with intravenous abuse of buprenorphine (Megarbane et al. 2006). As well as the overall greater safety there is also not the risk in titrating up quite quickly at the start of treatment to a therapeutically adequate dose, as there is with methadone. The subjective effects are less reinforcing than those of methadone, and the withdrawal symptoms from the drug itself are milder (Bickel & Amass 1995). This latter difference has had enormous impact in clinical practice, with patients often wishing to switch from methadone to buprenorphine for the final stages of a slow detoxification, to avoid methadone's own particular withdrawal effects, or indeed choosing to avoid methadone in the first place. In this chapter we will mainly refer to studies of buprenorphine as a maintenance treatment, and then its use in detoxification is presented in Chapter 3.

As with the sooner establishment of a sufficient therapeutic dose, another benefit of treatment which occurs more readily with buprenorphine than with methadone is the opiate-blocking effect. It is well known that full 'narcotic blockade' can occur with methadone but this does require exceptionally high-dose treatment, whereas the very ordinary dose of 16mg per day of buprenorphine produces about an 85% blocking effect on other opiates which may be taken, with this becoming nearly complete as doses go up from there (Greenwald et al. 2003). This is something else which is often greatly valued by users, who tend to think that this medication will help them better avoid the temptation of heroin. The aspect of quicker transfer to naltrexone after detoxification is discussed in the next chapter, and in the section on treating pregnant addicts the evidence is indicated showing less neonatal opioid withdrawal effect after treatment in pregnancy with buprenorphine than with methadone.

Use

For those of us in countries where buprenorphine and methadone are absolutely direct alternatives, with very broadly about half of presenting patients choosing one medication and half the other, there are two characteristics of the literature on buprenorphine from other countries which strike unusual notes. For anyone reviewing this area they will soon notice that an exceptional proportion of the literature comes from France (e.g. Auriacombe et al. 1999, Carrieri et al. 2006), and this is because even though buprenorphine use in substitution treatment there is recent, as it is everywhere else, methadone had not been widely used before it. Buprenorphine therefore attracted all the clearly advantageous study findings in routine treatment that other countries had when methadone was first introduced, while a further consideration in France has been that buprenorphine has mainly been used in the less secure and specialized settings such as primary care, and methadone in specialist centres.

Rather similar to this last point, the literature from the USA on buprenorphine sometimes reads as if this is a treatment for a different population to those who receive methadone. There are many references to 'the new heroin addicts', 'middle-class addicts' and treatment in 'office practice' for those who would not go to methadone clinics (e.g. Mitka 2003), with again sometimes less secure dispensing arrangements being required with buprenorphine.

There are a few echoes of these differences in countries such as the UK, and reference has been made elsewhere to the greater acceptability of buprenorphine by some patients who have become dependent on opioids through use in pain or even exercise regimes in combination with steroids, rather than through 'street' heroin. On the whole though these two main alternative treatments are both offered in routine clinical practice, with methadone perhaps being favoured for the more heavily addicted users. A patient's previous experience with the drugs either in or out of treatment can have a major bearing, although if illicit buprenorphine has been used in an uninformed way, for instance with precipitation of withdrawal with the first dose, some education can often be required before it is selected as a treatment. There is also a growing tendency for buprenorphine to be tried first in systematic treatment, as it is easier to transfer from this to methadone than the other way round.

Some study evidence

Buprenorphine was quickly found to be superior to placebo in opioid dependence, with a Cochrane review finding this to be so at high and very high doses of buprenorphine in all main aspects, with retention being superior even at definitely sub-therapeutic doses (Mattick et al. 2004). In Sweden Kakko et al. (2003) found that against a 'placebo' of just a 6-day medication reduction course the retention rate in buprenorphine treatment was 75% at 12 months, and with placebo was 0% at 2 months, with furthermore four deaths by 12 months in the latter group. The standard comparison in studies has become that with methadone, with the same Cochrane review being one of the influential papers to find that dosing in each group is crucial. Already there was evidence from a multicentre randomized trial that 8 mg per day of buprenorphine produced far better outcomes than the subtherapeutic 1 mg (Ling et al. 1998), while in another randomized study Mattick et al. (2004) considered that their slightly less good results from buprenorphine compared to methadone could have been due to too-slow induction. In the countries where buprenorphine and methadone tend to be given to different types of patients and in separate settings, the comparative studies have probably reflected features of the populations rather than true differences in effectiveness in some cases (e.g. Barrau et al. 2001), but a meta-analysis found high doses of methadone to be more effective than low doses of buprenorphine for retention rates and reductions in illicit opioid use, but similar to buprenorphine when that was in high dosage (Farre et al. 2002). In a study in Switzerland (Petitjean et al. 2001) some remarkably similar results between methadone and buprenorphine were found, such as 59% and 62% respectively in proportions of opioid-positive urine results and a similar pattern for cocaine, while in the light of subsequent clinical experience it is interesting that in a flexible dosing procedure mean stabilization doses were 10.5 mg per day for buprenorphine, and 69.8 mg per day for methadone.

It has been known for a long time that buprenorphine can satisfactorily be taken on alternate days, in double dosing (Amass et al. 1994), and indeed experiments in this way have been taken to the point of five or six times the daily maintenance dose every 120 hours (Gross et al. 2001)! Such extremes are not used in practice, but in some of the studies already mentioned it was apparently straightforward for dosing to be alternate-day. This therefore does have advantages in patients who are required to attend for supervised consumption, in the same way that it seemed that LAAM could be even more advantageous before that was withdrawn (see above). In the UK the vast majority of buprenorphine patients still take the drug daily, with the most obvious indication for trying the double-dosing being to avoid a take-home amount at weekends.

Particular practicalities

An excellent brief article on buprenorphine treatment has been provided by Taikato et al. (2005), which notes the common possible side-effects (headaches, nausea and vomiting, sweating, constipation, etc.) and drug interactions. The limited central depressant effect of buprenorphine may be compounded by alcohol and antidepressants, while the metabolism of buprenorphine can be enhanced by anticonvulsants, with therefore possibly reduced efficacy. There have been some case reports of liver toxicity from buprenorphine that is reversible if the medication is stopped (Herve et al. 2004), and often clinical guidelines will recommend that liver function tests are included in buprenorphine treatment, as they definitely should be with naltrexone.

The issue of starting dose of buprenorphine and how rapidly to increase has already been referred to, with probably inadequate induction being a recurrent theme in discussions within studies. It is common in practice for the first day's dose to be lower than that for the second day and ongoing, partly as any precipitated withdrawal will be less if adequate time since the last time of taking opiate has not passed. This is of the order of 12–16 hours after heroin and 24–36 hours after methadone, and rather than give a patient the tablets to take when such time has gone by it is preferable for a worker to be present then and double-check that they are actually in withdrawal. In the relatively demanding cases of transfer from methadone, therefore with a longer wait, some clinicians will 'bridge the gap' with a few days of low-dose diazepam or a (preferably non-benzodiazepine) sleeping tablet, and/or lofexidine, perhaps running into the first two days of taking the buprenorphine, when patients can feel quite unwell. A systematic study by Glasper et al. (2005) observed that it is common practice for patients to be required to be at the relatively low dose of 30 mg per day or so of methadone before switching to buprenorphine, and actually tested responses of methadone-dependent individuals going to buprenorphine from between 30 and 70 mg of methadone per day. Adjunctive lofexidine was prescribed, and the buprenorphine dose when transferred was 12–16 mg per day. There were no major differences found in difficulty of transfer between patients at the upper and lower ends of methadone dosage, although there was much support available as this was in an inpatient setting.

An issue which sometimes arises in practice, and can even be problematic enough to deter patients from switching from methadone to buprenorphine, is whether to apply the standard supervised consumption regime usually recommended when on a new medication. In many services the patients who will be changed in this way will almost by definition be progressing well in methadone treatment, in terms of avoiding other drugs, and may well have been allowed to have, say, twice-a-week collection of their medication. In the usual way therefore that precedents once set can be strongly held onto, such a patient may be very reluctant to go to daily supervised consumption 'just' because it is a different medication, and flexibility in this regard can be required.

Suboxone

Reference has already been made to the issue of diversion of buprenorphine, which is strongly related to the wish of some addicts to have this for injection (Jenkinson et al. 2005). In the UK, when buprenorphine is issued widely on a take-home basis a substantial degree of diversion does occur, with extraordinarily high prices being paid for tablets which find their way into prisons. Take-home policies are undoubtedly less problematic if the buprenorphine is given in the form of a combination tablet with naloxone, which has been gradually introduced following its development over a decade ago (Chapleo & Walter 1997). There is probably no strong reason why all buprenorphine given for unsupervised consumption should not be the combination product, at least to those who will not be pregnant, although at the time of writing the pharmaceutical committee in one of the areas where I work is objecting to a medication (naloxone) being given 'unnecessarily'. The rationale of the product is well-known and highly ingenious: if the patient takes their buprenorphine-naloxone tablet sublingually as they are meant to do they will just experience the buprenorphine, as naloxone is virtually inactive by that route, whereas if they abuse it by injection the antagonist effect will come into play as that is naloxone's active route. Undoubtedly some patients are reluctant to switch from standard buprenorphine to the combination product, but as noted at various stages in this book there is a strong link between 'acceptability' and abuse liability in the population whom we see. The pharmacological status of the combined medication has been well reviewed by Walsh and Eissenberg (2003).

Topic in brief – 6. Buprenorphine

- Is the main alternative to methadone, used just as much in many areas
- Has several advantages, including safety and less severe symptoms in withdrawal
- Opiate-blocking effect is more direct than with methadone and is valued by some patients
- Is seen in the USA as being largely for a different addict population in 'office practice', but this distinction is less in other countries
- The combination preparation with naloxone ingeniously deters injected abuse

---

Dihydrocodeine

Dihydrocodeine has had some appeal in drug-misuse treatment circles for a long time, as a medication which can be useful in substitution treatment, perhaps mainly in tapering dosage as a detoxification, with seemingly less severity of withdrawal symptoms than occurs from methadone. There has been much use of codeine and dihydrocodeine in this way in Germany, and positive results in maintenance treatment have been described, for instance by Krausz et al. (1998). There has also been something of a tradition of its use in Edinburgh in the UK, with staff from a specialized general practice treatment service there finding very favourable outcomes in an audit of 200 patients over several years (MacLeod et al. 1998). In a further study from the same area Robertson et al. (2006) found no significant differences in either retention or a range of standard drug-misuse outcome measures between patients randomized to methadone or dihydrocodeine.

Against this, however, many doctors have a highly negative view of dihydrocodeine because of the ease with which it can be given out in primary care – or any other medical setting for that matter – without the security requirements which apply to higher-level controlled drugs, with 'street' usage of dihydrocodeine very common. Also the place which dihydrocodeine perhaps used to occupy, i.e. between methadone and the use of non-opioid medications mainly for withdrawal, has in recent years been firmly taken by buprenorphine, with general acknowledgement that this again has less withdrawal severity than methadone. In many countries use of dihydrocodeine is now more discouraged, although no doubt it will continue to have its proponents.

Indeed, it is the very lack of the high security measures which apply to buprenorphine and methadone, plus the complications of buprenorphine, being sublingual and requiring overt withdrawal before taking the first dose, that partly explain the popularity of dihydrocodeine in some settings. It undoubtedly has a good degree of effectiveness in alleviating withdrawal features, and in the UK it is very commonly used to manage addicts who present for instance in police custody. This is basically in detoxification courses, and such usage is discussed a little further in Chapter 3.

Amphetamines

As indicated at the start of the chapter, there is some support for the view that the model of substitute prescribing which is used for opiate misusers should be extended to users of amphetamine. The availability of methadone enables treatment to be much more realistic by avoiding the requirement to be completely free of all opioid drugs, and the restriction of such an approach to users of one drug type can be viewed as both artificial and inequitable. The positive effect of methadone or alternative opioids on attraction into treatment is obvious, and it is argued that this effect is particularly needed in amphetamine users, who are generally a younger group but who are at significant risk of major psychiatric and physical complications (Klee 1992). In the UK amphetamine use is extremely common, and it has mainly been the HIV harm-reduction agenda which produced calls for a look at prescribing amphetamines, although not any other non-opiate drugs. So how suitable is it to offer such an option?

There are proportionally far more occasional and recreational users of amphetamine than of heroin, and so it would seem only relevant to apply the prescribing parallel at the heavier end of amphetamine usage. Even so, the conventional view is that since amphetamine is not a drug of true physical dependence, there is not the same requirement to intervene with a substitute to break the cycle whereby a drug is necessarily taken to avoid withdrawal symptoms. (The contrary view is that the emphasis on physical, meaning bodily, symptoms is unsatisfactory now that we appreciate the neurochemical basis for so-called psychological withdrawal features.) Also conventionally, amphetamine is seen as an inherently more destabilizing drug, with its stimulant effect and risk of psychosis, and so with these properties is not suitable to prescribe. Even if those objections are overcome, there is not a form of amphetamine which is long-acting, one of the benefits of methadone or buprenorphine for heroin users. Nevertheless, the contrast between treatments received by opiate and amphetamine users is stark, and the success of opioid maintenance, at the very least in engaging drug misusers, is such that some clinicians are attracted to experimentation with amphetamine prescribing. Certainly in clinical practice one encounters some daily users of large amounts of injected amphetamine who appear dependent in any meaningful sense of the word, and have the adverse social consequences which effectively represent much of the rationale for prescribing a substitute to heroin users. It is notable that such users typically do not appear excessively stimulated by amphetamine, but rather they are agitated at times of withdrawal, as if a paradoxical effect may be at work.

Fleming and Roberts (1994) reported the results of a small-scale experiment with amphetamine prescribing over three years in a UK clinic. Acceptance criteria included at least six months' daily injecting of the drug, and subjects received 30 mg of dexamphetamine sulphate per day in liquid form. The prescribed courses did not necessarily reduce, with two-thirds of the total subjects still receiving prescriptions at the time of reporting, at a mean duration of 15 months. Medication consumption was supervised, and there were compulsory group meetings aimed at enhancing motivation and advising on harm reduction. With this approach over half the subjects were apparently able to stop injecting, as confirmed by physical examination, and there were substantial reductions in injecting by the remainder. There were consequent reductions in HIV-risk behaviours, although sexual practices were largely unchanged. The anticipated increase in amphetamine users presenting for treatment did occur. The authors observed that their results might have been even better had they prescribed higher doses of dexamphetamine; their calculation, which took into account the very low purity and presence of active and inactive forms in street amphetamine, was based on a street usage of 1 g per day, but probably most daily injectors use more than that.

A report of similar treatment came from Victoria, Australia, also with encouraging results (Sherman 1990). A group of 14 street amphetamine addicts, mostly injectors, were prescribed 20–90 mg of dexamphetamine sulphate per day, with a substance administered to alkalinize the urine to prolong the half-life of the drug. Stabilization followed by slow reduction was the aim and, although treatment became prolonged in some cases, others apparently remained drug-free after their reducing course. As with many areas of experimental prescribing, however, most experience has been in the UK, where the extent to which this option has been tried is perhaps surprising in that it has gone against very clear advisory guidance. Guidelines on clinical management of drug misuse issued by the Department of Health to all doctors (Department of Health 1991) stated simply that 'it is undesirable to prescribe substitute stimulant drugs as the risk of them being misused is very high'. Nevertheless, at a time when those were the current guidelines, Strang and Sheridan (1997b) estimated from a survey of community pharmacies that approximately a thousand addicts were receiving amphetamine prescriptions. Only 8% of prescriptions were from private practice, and nearly half were from general practitioners.

The views and clinical practice of drug-misuse specialists in the UK in relation to amphetamine prescribing were surveyed in the same period (Bradbeer et al. 1998), with, remarkably, 60% of 149 respondents considering that this approach had a place in clinical management. Forty-six per cent of the responding specialists did actually prescribe amphetamine, with others who approved in principle, but did not do so, giving lack of experience or budget limitations as their reasons. The main reasons for not approving

Table 2.2 Features of amphetamine prescribing by drug misuse specialists in the UK

Criteria
Long-term use
Injecting
No mental illness
Prescription
Dexamphetamine tablets or suspension
20–200 mg/day
Not time-limited
Monitoring
Urine
Injection sites
Location
More outside London

Based on Bradbeer et al. (1998)

of prescribing were a lack of evidence to say that it helps, risk of psychosis, no physical addiction, and budget limitations. The survey included some details of prescribing policies, and Table 2.2 indicates the features which emerged as something of a consensus.

Prescribing was mainly considered for long-term amphetamine injectors, and half the respondents also required absence of mental illness as a criterion. Dexamphetamine sulphate tablets were prescribed more than the suspension, at a mean maximum dose of 66 mg per day, while one clinician was giving injectable amphetamine ampoules. Two-thirds of prescribers did not set a time limit on the period for which individuals could receive prescriptions, with monitoring apparently nearly always by urine screening and examination of injection sites. In practice, the latter is particularly useful in this group, as the committed long-term injectors for whom prescribing is considered are typically reluctant to use street amphetamine in any other way. Also, a special urinalysis technique has been described which largely enables separate identification of prescribed dex-amphetamine and street amphetamine, by measuring the isomer ratio of d-amphetamine, which is present in both, to l-amphetamine, which is in the street preparation only (Tetlow & Merrill 1996).

Since the studies mentioned so far there has continued to be interest in amphetamine substitute prescribing, with some encouraging results but crucially little support from a randomized controlled trial. In a case-control study Klee et al. (2001) found that amphetamine misusers prescribed dexamphetamine tended to be making better progress than similar users not offered that approach, and one case-note investigation even indicated that dexamphetamine could unproblematically be given to dual diagnosis patients with schizophrenia and amphetamine dependence (Carnwath et al. 2002). The aspect mentioned above of being able to separately distinguish use of illicit amphetamines from the prescribed form in the urine has been considered important, with further work carried out in this area

(George & Braithwaite 2000). However, something of a 'nail in the coffin' of amphetamine prescribing, which has always been unpopular with advisory authorities, was ironically provided by a controlled study carried out by specialists who had otherwise been advocates of the policy (Merrill et al. 2005). The intervention of prescribing dexamphetamine, for a four-month period before reducing the dose to zero, and initially at a maximum of 100 mg per day, was compared to standard treatment without prescribing, with ratings at various key stages and then a nine-month follow-up. Although both groups showed reductions in injecting and illicit amphetamine use there was no significant difference between them, with the main benefits for amphetamine prescribing seemingly restricted to some of the health measures at some points.

It does seem as if these results have contributed to a currently more negative climate towards prescribing; after the simple recommendation not to do this in early Department of Health guidelines mentioned above, the advice became slightly more encouraging in an intervening set (Department of Health 1999), but the latest version of this guidance for doctors in the UK (Department of Health 2007) states that although there was 'previously thought to be a limited place for the prescription of dexamphetamine [which] still occurs in some parts of the UK ... substitute stimulant prescribing does not have demonstrated effectiveness and, accordingly, should not ordinarily be provided'. Perhaps the word 'ordinarily' is key, as virtually no one considers that amphetamine prescribing should be at all routine, whereas many services have a very few individuals of the type described at the start of this section for whom the prescribing option is at least considered.

Even where prescribing does occur it is often limited in duration, with cessation or gradual reduction occurring in a way that is increasingly considered unwise with opiate prescribing. There is actually no very strong reason to believe that relapse will occur less in the kinds of amphetamine users for whom prescribing is done than it would for opiate users, and it seems that the limitations in what is given have more to do with the anyway uncertain status of amphetamine prescribing as an option. When such withdrawal does take place it can be done either by cuts in the daily dosage, or by progressively omitting days in a week from the prescription, therefore somewhat mimicking recreational usage. In practice there is also some concern that the risk of psychosis and mood disturbances could be increased if the pure prescribed form of amphetamine is continued, although this is not much backed by the reports of progress in studies.

Case history

Peter is 46 years old, married with two children. He has been using amphetamines for 30 years, starting at a time when pharmaceutical amphetamines and barbiturates were prominent in the illicit drug scene, at nightclubs. In the early years he also abused pharmaceutical opioids, and he has continued to have cannabis and alcohol regularly. He went through a period of undoubted alcohol dependence, but throughout his 'career' his favoured drug has been amphetamine.

Following earlier occasional contacts Peter was referred to our service a year ago, largely as a result of his wife's concerns. Both she and Peter felt that a lifestyle change was required, and that the needs of their teenage children were being neglected. Peter's usage of amphetamine had gradually increased to about 7 g per day, injecting about six times per 24 hours. After each injection he would go to his bedroom and listen to loud 'rave' music for hours, and his wife was exasperated that he generally did very little else. Some evenings he would also go on to nightclubs, where he would use ecstasy.

Treatment aimed at short-term cessation of amphetamine use was considered completely unrealistic. After the necessary discussions the substitution prescribing option was initiated, with the harm-reduction objective of at least reducing Peter's injecting and use of street amphetamine. He was given dexamphetamine sulphate liquid 60 mg per day, with a plan to reduce gradually over the following months.

Treatment has been very successful, with a remarkable change in Peter's behaviour. Regular examination of injecting sites confirms his and his wife's reports of a dramatic decline in street amphetamine use, with many benefits for their domestic situation. Finances have greatly improved, the children's needs are being attended to, and they are to take a family holiday. Peter's behaviour is generally much more appropriate, and for the first time in years he is helping his wife in house duties. Although he had not been prone to psychosis, he had previously had much mood disturbance on street amphetamine, and his mood state has also greatly improved.

Because of the benefits we have not imposed a rapid reduction, with just two incremental reductions to 50 mg per day. However, we have gradually introduced amphetamine-free days, and his prescription is now for only four days each week.

Benzodiazepines

I shall start by declaring that in our clinical services we find issues to do with benzodiazepines some of the most frequent causes of disagreement with patients, probably second only to reimbursement of bus fares to attend the clinic. Patients on benefits do indeed receive such funds if they can show tickets but this seems not always straightforward to do, and when I mentioned in a case conference recently that our disputes always seemed to be about 'bus fares and benzos', one of the local professors suggested that could be a title for the book!

Looking at the matter very broadly, the problem is that a possible benzodiazepine misuser attending clinic knows that their drug is something that could be prescribed to them, in contrast to other polydrug users whose preference is for cocaine, cannabis or another street preparation. It might be thought that the parallel with methadone or buprenorphine for heroin addicts is reasonable, but on the contrary benzodiazepines are nearly always a secondary drug of misuse and there is often far more question about the presence of any actual dependence, with virtually no support for 'maintenance' prescribing in any national guidelines. If too much of a benzodiazepine 'culture' gets going in a drug clinic a situation occurs where a daytime tranquillizer and a sleeping tablet become almost routine 'side orders' along with the main opioid, and even the most casual examination indicates that many of the benzodiazepines will travel far away from the person to whom they were given. To add to the sources of dispute, illicit drug users often take doses far in excess of the therapeutic regimes that are approved for short-term use, in for instance the British National Formulary (2008) (Seivewright 1998, Nielsen et al. 2007).

If a very strict line is taken against any benzodiazepine prescribing to drug misusers in a specialist clinic different problems can occur. I have worked covering districts where the local specialist has laid down that they will prescribe no benzodiazepines in their opioid clinic, and that any such prescribing needs to be done in general practice. The primary care setting, however, is undoubtedly even more exploitable in this respect than a clinic used to preventing early collecting and indeed having drugs on daily supervised consumption (daily dispensing of diazepam from a community pharmacy is now legislated for in the UK), and in our own services we feel that if anybody is to be involved with prescribing benzodiazepines the dependence clinic ought to be able to address the matter most securely and satisfactorily.

In view of the potential pitfalls in giving benzodiazepines to polydrug users, the subject will be examined carefully, starting with probably the only situation in which it is definitely advisable to prescribe, which is in short-term withdrawal from benzodiazepine misuse where there is demonstrable physical dependence and within a closely monitored arrangement.

Detoxification from benzodiazepine misuse

In this indication, the most important clinical consideration is determining what level of treatment is required. The answer seems to be, not as much as might be expected from the evidence relating to ordinary low-dose usage. Since it was demonstrated that physical dependence on benzodiazepines could occur in a proportion of cases (Tyrer et al. 1981), individuals who have become dependent after prescription for minor psychiatric disorders are typically offered reducing courses of benzodiazepines lasting several months or more (Lader & Morton 1991, Oude Voshaar et al. 2006). To adopt the equivalent approach in drug misusers, with conversions for the far higher dosages that many of this group consume, would be quite unmanageable and inadvisable, and the first reason to avoid this is that not all benzodiazepine misusers become physically dependent. We demonstrated (Seivewright & Dougal 1993) that polydrug users in situations of stopping benzodiazepines can experience classic benzodiazepine withdrawal symptoms, in our study more severe after high dosage, multiple benzodiazepine use, and oral rather than injected use. With regard to the *proportion* of polydrug users who develop such symptoms, Williams et al. (1996) found in a detoxification unit that benzodiazepine withdrawal symptoms emerged in less than half of opiate addicts reporting current benzodiazepine misuse. Furthermore, in that study the dose of diazepam required for stabilization in those who did exhibit withdrawal features was unrelated to claimed previous benzodiazepine usage, at a mean dose of 40 mg per day.

This low level of prescribing is supported by the findings, at an early stage, of Harrison et al. (1984), that in 23 individuals who had previously used a mean diazepam equivalent of 140 mg per day, diazepam detoxification starting at 40% of reported daily consumption, followed by daily tapering by 10%, ensured satisfactory completion in most cases. Also, a reduction from 60 mg of diazepam over six days has specifically been claimed to avoid convulsions in benzodiazepine misusers who had previously had that complication (Scott 1990). Given the high incidence of secondary benzodiazepine misuse among addicts there has been remarkably little study of withdrawal schemes, with a recent systematic review observing that all controlled studies of benzodiazepine detoxification excluded subjects who were on opiates (Fatseas et al. 2006). From other kinds of studies, however, the authors were still able to conclude that 'the best evidence supports a procedure where the patient is switched to a long-lasting benzodiazepine and the dose then tapered by 25% of the initial dose each week', therefore again supporting quick timescales. In inpatient units withdrawal schemes can safely be even more rapid (McGregor et al. 2003), and can sometimes involve the anticonvulsants carbamazepine or sodium valproate rather than benzodiazepines themselves (Kristensen et al. 2006).

Other benzodiazepine prescribing

A huge amount of unsatisfactory prescribing of benzodiazepines to drug misusers is encountered, including situations where they appear to be given as little more than a token gesture, to provide some satisfaction without the complications of issuing specific treatments such as methadone. Guidance on such matters is an important role for drug services, and also the precedents set by our own prescribing must always be borne in mind. Although in various situations we may see a case for some prescribing of benzodiazepines, such prescribing to polydrug users can in one way make it more difficult for us to advise others not to do this.

One emerging usage of short-term benzodiazepines is in states characterized by agitation, such as withdrawal states in stimulant users. In a survey of treatment of cocaine misuse in England, we found that over 10% of services had recently prescribed benzodiazepines to primary cocaine users, in a range of clinical situations (Seivewright et al. 2000a). Withdrawal from heavy use of crack cocaine provides a good example of the need to weigh the possible benefits of benzodiazepines in reducing agitation and withdrawal distress against the risk of erratic usage in an unstable situation, and the problems of establishing a precedent, including sometimes introducing a user to a new medication of misuse. There is also the concern that benzodiazepines may paradoxically increase aggressiveness, a phenomenon which is often quoted although the actual evidence is not strong (Bond 1993). This is potentially important in drug misusers, who as a group have high rates of aggressive and impulsive behaviours, but there is a suggestion from animal experiments with benzodiazepines that the aggression-enhancing effect occurs in those whose basal levels are relatively low (Mos & Oliver 1987).

Case history

Carl is a 25-year-old man who was referred urgently and presented to the clinic along with his mother. He had been using crack cocaine for two years, and it was apparent that he had previously been a dealer in this drug. This was in the context of a generally criminal lifestyle, with previous convictions for armed robbery. He said that when initially dealing in the drug he 'never touched it myself', but that now he had a substantial crack habit. He used the drug compulsively with extreme craving, and gave the example of obtaining a financial loan to buy a car and then spending all the money in two days on crack. A urine drug screen confirmed use of cocaine, and there was evidence of related instability of mood, with Carl breaking down in tears in the assessment appointments. His mother was extremely distressed and told us that Carl had stolen and sold most of the valuable family possessions.

Residential treatment appeared the most likely way of making an impact on Carl's crack cocaine use, and plans were made for an admission. This could not happen immediately, and in the meantime Carl was prescribed fluoxetine 20 mg per day, and diazepam 20–30 mg per day. He was keen to try to withdraw himself from crack without going into hospital, and he and his mother were instructed about his use of the two medications. They were advised that diazepam would reduce anxiety and agitation, and might help relieve craving for crack.

One week later Carl told us that he had managed to completely avoid crack use, which was supported by urine sampling. His mother said that he had appeared drowsy on the diazepam, a medication which he had not had before, while Carl reported a generally helpful calming effect. He had also taken the fluoxetine, and there was a suggestion of a reduction in depression. After another week the situation was similar, although with the sedative effects of diazepam less marked. Carl felt that he did not need inpatient treatment as he had been able to stop using crack in this way, but unfortunately after that he dropped out of outpatient contact with us.

Benzodiazepines obtained by illicit drug users are no doubt put to a range of uses, of varying drug-related harm. The implications of controlled usage in opiate misusers in treatment are considered below, and in the discussions on opiate detoxification. Gossop et al. (1991) found that addicts in opiate withdrawal treatment had frequently used benzodiazepines in attempts at self-detoxification; this may arguably be seen as constructive use, but it may have been very uncontrolled and, given the setting, the attempts had clearly not been ultimately successful. Benzodiazepines appear to provide nonspecific relief in withdrawal from virtually any drug, including opiates (Drummond et al. 1989), but in practical terms it is only satisfactory to prescribe them for that purpose as part of a structured detoxification package.

Prescribing benzodiazepines to opioid substitution patients

This is a controversial area which arises frequently in the UK. Greenwood (1996) published results from the clinical treatment service in Edinburgh, in which impressive reductions in overall illicit drug use and drug injecting had been achieved with a prescribing policy which included benzodiazepines alongside methadone in two-thirds of cases. In the earlier influential studies which provided such strong support for the original model of methadone maintenance there was no benzodiazepine prescribing but, as we observed in Chapter 1, these often excluded individuals with polydrug use. Multiple drug use is now often the norm in those presenting for opioid treatment, and strategies to address substantial degrees of benzodiazepine misuse are increasingly required. This is partly as benzodiazepines are certainly given very frequently to opiate-dependent patients: in a postal survey Williams et al. (2005) found that three-quarters of responding drug services were prescribing benzodiazepines to opioid patients for detoxification and 35% for benzodiazepine maintenance, even though general practitioners were noted to be one of the most common sources of benzodiazepines. There are very few controlled studies of additional benzodiazepine prescribing to guide us, and so for the present the subject must largely be approached from a clinical perspective. In Table 2.3 I have attempted an analysis of the pros and cons of prescribing benzodiazepines in any more than the short term to drug misusers, the usual clinical situation in which this arises being ongoing methadone or buprenorphine treatment.

One indication for prescription of benzodiazepines may be in individuals who are considered simply too dependent to withdraw successfully, just as is the case with a minority of ordinary-dose users. In such cases it is extremely important to restrict benzodiazepine consumption to the clinic's own supplies, and indeed one reason why a clinic may undertake some benzodiazepine prescribing is to be able to seal off other sources of supply, for instance from general practitioners. Different models of medical provision across countries mean that this is easier to achieve in some areas than others, and in general there is probably more sympathy for clinic benzodiazepine prescribing in systems where stopping other prescribing is relatively straightforward. Critics can point to the fallibility of such arrangements, the availability of benzodiazepines in the street drug scene, and the particular limitations of urine drug screening in separately identifying the different benzodiazepines.

Table 2.3 Rationales for and against prescribing long-term benzodiazepines to drug misusers

For	Against
Some users too dependent to stop	Promotes dependence
Control existing benzodiazepine usage	Risk of erratic or dangerous usage
May enable avoidance of street drugs	Benzodiazepine use associated with worse outcomes in some studies
Effective symptomatic treatment in individuals with poor coping resources	Prescribing can set unsatisfactory precedent

More fundamentally in terms of clinical progress, some methadone or buprenorphine patients appear to be able to stop using street drugs, notably heroin, if their prescription is augmented by benzodiazepines, when they have not previously been able to stop on the opioid alone. It is possible to contend that in such circumstances patients have been on inadequate opioid doses, but clinically this does not always seem a sufficient explanation. The so-called 'opiate-enhancing' property of benzodiazepines probably produces a different effect to that of simply more methadone (Preston et al. 1984, Bell et al. 1990), and while in services we generally do not wish to encourage drug combinations or 'dual dependency', taking the two drugs may be reasonably satisfactory in some cases. In many ways the issues for the prescriber are similar to those in stepping up to injectable methadone or an alternative more euphoriant opioid, always with the purpose of stopping street drug use; in this instance some individuals may have been taking heroin or cannabis to get to sleep, which benzodiazepines can replace. We also often encounter the situation of patients positively wishing to manage on a lower dose of methadone or buprenorphine and, as discussed previously, we will not always stand in the way of this, even given the disadvantage of adding benzodiazepines. Finally, in terms of possible grounds for prescribing, the efficacy of benzodiazepines in treating anxiety and insomnia is readily appreciated by individuals who are not 'psychologically minded', and have poor coping resources, and some clinicians may accept such a situation if they can take steps to see that misuse is not occurring.

Against prescribing, it seems inherently unsatisfactory in a drug dependence clinic to prescribe benzodiazepines with a regularity which may induce dependence, especially if this is not directly a response to previous benzodiazepine misuse. However, philosophically this is something of a dilemma: dependence (rather than adverse effects) has been identified as the main problem for ordinary-dose licit benzodiazepine users but, in comparison with that group, if a drug misuser is already dependent on 80 mg of methadone per day is it more, or less, of an issue that they may become dependent on benzodiazepines? More practically, the risk of erratic usage is ever-present, particularly where the prescription systems which enable daily dispensing of opioid treatment cannot stipulate this for benzodiazepines. The over-use of larger supplies has to be continually guarded against, with the worst consequence being fatality from combined drug misuse. As discussed in Chapter 1, studies of individuals who have died taking methadone show benzodiazepines and other sedatives such as alcohol to be frequently implicated, and although the majority of such deaths involve outright abuse of methadone, the addition of benzodiazepines to a prescribed regime clearly increases the overall direct risk. The situation is even more clear-cut with buprenorphine, in which fatal overdose is seemingly not possible from correct use of the drug alone, but can be if benzodiazepines are also involved (Reynaud et al. 1998, Megarbane et al. 2006).

A series of studies in Sydney (Darke et al. 1992b, 1993, 1994a) found that benzodiazepine use in illicit drug users was associated with various adverse features, including poor physical and psychological health, more injecting, HIV-risk behaviours and polydrug use, and worse social impairment, although these were not studies of individuals prescribed benzodiazepines as part of a methadone programme. It should be noted that a very similar list of correlates is found in drug misusers who have personality disorder (Darke et al. 1994b, Seivewright & Daly 1997) – it may well be that the two aspects are related (King et al. 2001), or generally that benzodiazepine use tends to be an indicator of the more problematic cases of drug misuse. An important practical point in weighing the benefits and risks of issuing benzodiazepines to opioid patients is that any prescribing sets a precedent, in which benzodiazepines may be dubiously claimed as an entitlement when a patient presents elsewhere. As indicated above, this also applies in other prescribing situations, and such claims can be extremely troublesome in clinical practice. In our clinics we have taken the decision to issue no further prescriptions for temazepam to newly presenting patients, partly because of the unfortunate example which prescribing sets, even though it might possibly be justified in some individual cases. It can be argued that the particular problems resulting from injected abuse of temazepam (see Chapter 4) are less likely now that the capsules with liquid contents are unavailable, but the drug is still unduly sought after by illicit drug users and injection undoubtedly still occurs, and we feel that the benefits of avoiding such prescribing outweigh any limitations. It is made clear to patients that there are simply no exceptions to this rule, and we have had no significant problems in implementing the policy over a decade or so.

If an opioid maintenance patient does receive benzodiazepines, the implications for their treatment contract should be as if they had injectable methadone or a more euphoriant opioid, although arguably the expectations may not be quite as high. The basic approach should be that since they have been given an additional medication with inherent disadvantages, probably because of an inability to stabilize on the opioid alone, they must show abstinence from street drugs, otherwise there is no point in giving the additional medication. In some UK clinics benzodiazepine prescribing is so widespread that this would unfortunately be seen as a counsel of perfection. The most justifiable reason for continuing a prescription of oral methadone plus benzodiazepines in the face of some ongoing drug misuse is if it effectively avoids the need for a higher-level type of prescription, in somebody who would otherwise be a candidate. A common such situation over the years has been where a persistent desire to use drugs by injection is reduced by benzodiazepines, enough to render an injectable prescription unnecessary, but not enough to result in complete cessation.

Finally, it should be stressed again that certainly not all benzodiazepine prescribing to opioid maintenance patients need be long term. McDuff et al. (1993) reported on detoxification from alprazolam, the benzodiazepine most commonly used by their methadone subjects. With methadone dosage usually remaining the same, patients were offered a set reducing course of alprazolam over 11 weeks. Of 22 patients, four refused the treatment and 12 out of 18 subsequently completed detoxification, although timescales in practice proved variable. In a comparative study by Weizman et al. (2003) just over a quarter of benzodiazepine-dependent methadone maintenance patients remained free of benzodiazepines after a systematic clonazepam withdrawal, although more success in avoiding illicit benzodiazepine use was found if the clonazepam was maintained. In practice, as opposed to set study protocols, it is easy to recognize that much prescribing of benzodiazepines intended to be short-term drifts into a more prolonged situation, which fits with analyses of prescribing in methadone clinics (Best et al. 2002).

Case history

Yousef is 27 years old and has been in methadone treatment for five years. He had previously used heroin for nearly as long, and initially in methadone treatment had found it very difficult to give up use of this drug. He would have heroin about once a week, with many urine samples positive and sanctions imposed at various stages. His other drug of preference was alcohol, and he would sometimes attend the clinic intoxicated. There were generally limited expectations of progress, and he had few other social opportunities, being unemployed with no qualifications. He had served one prison sentence and was regularly charged for being drunk and disorderly. He has always been very unenthusiastic about an increase in methadone, claiming to be quite comfortable on his 40 mg per day and to have other reasons for his heroin and alcohol use. He would drink in the daytime, not to alleviate withdrawal symptoms but more as a form of tranquillization, and about two years ago it was agreed that he could have some benzodiazepines prescribed to try and reduce his other drug use. It was made very clear that these would be stopped very quickly if there was no such improvement, and he was seen frequently during the early stages of benzodiazepine prescribing. After various adjustments his prescription stabilized at methadone 40 mg per day, diazepam 25 mg per day and limited (not continuous) zopiclone.

Although this approach is theoretically unsatisfactory, Yousef has proved able to avoid other drug use on the combination of methadone and moderate doses of benzodiazepines. He is never now intoxicated in clinic, and we have independent information that his drinking has greatly reduced. Most notably, all his monthly urine samples for well over a year have shown only methadone and benzodiazepines. He is regularly reminded that we are only prepared to give him benzodiazepines if we can see such clear progress, but he is adamant that this combination enables him to stop using other drugs.

Alternatives to benzodiazepines

In any of the clinical situations in drug misuse where a benzodiazepine may be used, the less addictive alternatives should be considered. These fall into two groups: medications which are known from established usage to have little misuse potential other than in exceptional individuals, and the newer alternatives to benzodiazepines, about which we can be less certain. In the first category, low doses of sedative antipsychotic drugs are sometimes used for agitation in stimulant users, particularly in inpatients, and in some settings they feature in opiate withdrawal regimes. They may be tried as management of anxiety or insomnia, provided doses are well below the threshold of neurological side-effects, or some clinicians will use low doses of the sedative antidepressants for sleeping problems. Trazodone provides sedation with the lowest level of antidepressant side-effects, with mirtazepine another possibility, while the least toxic option for night sedation is the antihistamine promethazine. The second category of medication includes buspirone for anxiety, and zopiclone and zolpidem for insomnia, all of which produce less physical dependence than the benzodiazepines but are unlikely to be completely free of related problems. Zopiclone in particular has been associated with daytime misuse (Hajak et al. 2003), and is perhaps the most similar to the benzodiazepines in overall effects. In our service we have seen some extraordinary cases of ultra-high-dose abuse of zolpidem, and such reports in the literature suggest a range of desired effects by users (Liappas et al. 2003).

While there are sound theoretical reasons for selecting these alternative medications, there is an ever-present problem of generally low acceptability in drug misusers, although this can definitely be changed to a degree by establishing a suitable culture of expectation within a clinic. Unfortunately some acceptability issues are quite inevitable, given the links between acceptability and misuse liability for this population, particularly the less well-motivated. Probably nearly all drug-misuse clinicians would agree that benzodiazepine prescribing should be kept as low as possible, but such true benefits as there are in a minority of cases no doubt partly depend on the particular agonist and subjective effects of those drugs. Also, as in low-dose users, the alternatives are ineffective where there are withdrawal symptoms in cases of established benzodiazepine dependence, and the main role for these medications in drug misusers would appear to be in attempts to avoid initial exposure to benzodiazepines.

Topic in brief – 7. Benzodiazepine prescribing to illicit drug users

- Should only be done if it is certainly not occurring from elsewhere
- Can be at much lower doses than reported usage
- Detoxification courses can safely be short
- Is only justified on an ongoing basis if it demonstrably enables cessation of illicit drug use
- Is unnecessary where safer and less addictive alternatives can be used

3

Treatments
Achieving detoxification and abstinence

Introduction

Whatever else a drug misuse treatment service does, it must be able to successfully withdraw individuals from addictive drugs. In recent years there has been much emphasis on methadone maintenance, partly on harm-reduction grounds, but meanwhile in the UK heroin has become readily available in most localities, and many users with short histories are presenting as suitable for detoxification treatments. In particular, young people are commonly turning to heroin after recreational use of amphetamine, ecstasy, LSD or cannabis, and are then often distressed by the development of physical dependence, which is in contrast to their previous drug experiences. A proportion of this group become committed heroin users, but many present for help to come off the drug, and typically do not want methadone or any other ongoing substitution treatment. Some drug services have found it difficult to adjust to this group of users, who may be reluctant to attend a place which they see as dominated by maintenance candidates, and who have very different treatment needs. In our services we consider the detoxification of young heroin users to be one of the main priorities in providing an effective community treatment response, and have gained much experience in this type of work. The first part of this chapter describes the methods we use for non-opioid community detoxifications, where we find that successful withdrawal can frequently be achieved, *provided* that much attention is paid both to patient selection and to organization in treatment.

Individuals who are more heavily dependent on opiates clearly also require detoxification at various stages, and the remainder of the chapter discusses other forms of withdrawal treatment. As indicated in Chapter 1, community detoxification with methadone, as opposed to maintenance, is not well supported by evidence, but nevertheless this has been a standard treatment in the UK and other countries for many years. Meanwhile the almost certainly milder withdrawal symptoms from buprenorphine make this a more attractive proposition than methadone in detoxification, and the major impact made recently by this treatment will be examined. The last section discusses relapse prevention, focusing on counselling approaches and on the use of the opiate antagonist naltrexone, which we recommend after most detoxifications from opiates.

Quick detoxifications from heroin

Assessment, preparation and level of support required

Quick detoxification is a concentrated treatment approach, which requires motivation and organization on the part of both the drug user and the drug team worker. It is important not to attempt the treatment in unsuitable cases, and selection must be based

Table 3.1 Features desirable for quick community detoxification from heroin

Short history
Low level of use
Not injecting
No significant current other drug use
Good motivation
Absence of personality disorder
Supportive family member(s) or partner to be involved

not simply on whether an individual is 'saying the right things', but on relatively objective aspects of their drug use and situation which can predict outcome. Our experience points to the features in Table 3.1 as indicating likely successful completion of quick detoxification treatment.

A short history of heroin use is definitely desirable, preferably not more than a year to 18 months. The level of usage should be reduced during preparation for detoxification, but ideally has not been more than a gram per day (locally approximately 20% pure) at its peak. Current injecting usually counts against this form of treatment, and such users may be offered an intervening period on buprenorphine or methadone so that they can give up injecting before having to give up opiate use; however, the population we see tend not to want methadone in particular, and some users can convert from injecting to smoking once supportive counselling is under way. Significant use of any other drug makes uncomplicated completion of quick detoxification from heroin unlikely, while heavy previous usage, for instance a history of daily injected use of amphetamine, may also be a poor prognostic sign. Crucially, individuals must be well-motivated, and free from significant personality disorder, which appears to exert a generally adverse effect in detoxification attempts (Seivewright & Daly 1997). Finally, it is highly preferable if there is a family member or drug-free partner in the household to be actively involved in the detoxification, in terms of helping to manage medication and reducing the possibility of drugs being obtained at times of problems. Sometimes a couple will do this form of detoxification together, but it is unlikely to work if one partner or anyone else in the household is still actively using.

We find that a brief stage of preparation for the detoxification pays dividends, and sometimes no medication is issued at the assessment appointment. A urine sample is taken for drug screening to confirm the history, and the user is advised in standard drug counselling terms regarding taking responsibility for their own drug use and monitoring it, methods of cutting down, dealing with triggers and high-risk situations, and the assertive tactics in relation to lifestyle and drug-using acquaintances which will be necessary in retracting from the drug scene. At one or more closely spaced appointments the worker assesses progress, and full detoxification starts when usage has reduced sufficiently, preferably to under a quarter of a gram per day.

Information on the withdrawal process is provided, along with schedules for the detoxification medications, and the treatment is also explained to anyone else who will be involved. Importantly, the detoxification takes place when the worker can fit in home visits through the period, preferably every day, and so it is not usually suitable to start a detoxification at a weekend. Given a well-organized service with competent drug workers, the only time a doctor need see the user is just prior to detoxification, to confirm that the method selected is suitable and to issue the prescription; the next involvement is to initiate naltrexone if detoxification has been successfully completed. This limited medical input can be provided either from the clinic, or by a user's general practitioner in liaison with the drug worker.

Method 1 – Symptomatic medication

Individuals on very small amounts of heroin are prescribed diazepam for anxiety, agitation or craving, zopiclone or zolpidem for insomnia, hyoscine butylbromide (Buscopan) for stomach cramps, and diphenoxylate/atropine (Lomotil) for diarrhoea, over a seven-day period. The medication schedule provided to the user explains which drug is for which symptoms, and the maximum doses of each that can be taken in a day, which for diazepam varies during the course. The basic medication regime is included in the Appendix.

Method 2 – Lofexidine plus symptomatic medication

This is our main method of quick detoxification from heroin, suitable for most individuals of the type described in the assessment section above. The symptomatic medication options remain the same, but the principal treatment is lofexidine, an analogue of clonidine which does not have that drug's hypotensive effect and is therefore entirely suitable for community treatment. As a non-opioid method of controlling opiate withdrawal symptoms, it is an inherently appealing treatment to use in heroin users not severe enough to require methadone, and in the UK it has been widely taken up by drug services for that indication. Since something of a peak of lofexidine use perhaps a decade ago, there has been the emergence of buprenorphine, which in the UK now occupies a large part of the 'middle ground' of the treatment range. Detoxification with buprenorphine is described later in the chapter, while lofexidine can be useful towards the end of a reducing course of that drug.

The evidence for effectiveness of lofexidine initially relied on the similarity with clonidine, without the same risk of hypotension, but there have increasingly been controlled studies of lofexidine itself (Bearn et al. 1996, Khan et al. 1997, Lin et al. 1997). The better toleration and somewhat broader effectiveness of lofexidine was demonstrated in a randomized study against clonidine (Gerra et al. 2001), while the need for some adjunctive medications is suggested by experimental studies (Walsh et al. 2003) as well as clinical experience.

In our protocol the lofexidine dosage increases and then gradually decreases over six days, being at its highest when heroin withdrawal symptoms would be expected to peak. The medication regime is indicated in the Appendix. The initial increase in dose is at a quicker rate than was recommended in the lofexidine (Britlofex) prescribing data sheet (Britannia Pharmaceuticals) when the medication was first licensed, but that document has since been revised upwards, more in line with much clinical usage which occurred. In an inpatient comparison with methadone, Bearn et al. (1996) used what were the standard incremental increases in lofexidine up to ten 0.2mg tablets per day, but considered that dosing to be probably suboptimal. More rapid increases are now commonplace and recommended, with another change in licensing in the UK being that lofexidine can be used for somewhat longer periods, i.e. more than 10 days. While studies show little or no reduction in blood pressure, occasionally suggestive symptoms such as faintness on standing up are encountered, with low-body-weight females possibly particularly susceptible. Blood pressure should be checked before treatment and can be retested at visits, or for self-monitoring we instruct patients to check their pulse before a lofexidine dose, and to omit that dose if it is below 60 beats per minute.

Case history

Lee is 19 and works for a sports equipment firm. From the age of 16 he had used cannabis, LSD, amphetamines and ecstasy, but he claimed that none of this use had been heavy. He would use amphetamine, orally, about once every two weeks, and he liked to have one ecstasy tablet if he went to a nightclub. Ecstasy is the drug he would most want to continue, although he has been made aware of the risks. He has always kept himself fit, and sees recreational drug use as a normal thing for his generation.

His problem over the past year has been heroin, on which he became dependent following initial experimental use. After about three months he would get withdrawal symptoms if he did not have the drug daily, and his usage stabilized at 0.5g per day, by smoking. He resented the control which heroin had gained over his life, and he could see that his general health was suffering. He told us 'I'm sick of heroin and I just want off it'.

Lee attended for a short series of counselling appointments to do the preparatory work for a detoxification. His parents had become aware of the problem, and after initial distress they were keen to help him through his treatment. With the counsellor's advice, Lee reduced his heroin use to the minimum which he needed to stop him withdrawing, and it was arranged that he had our standard detoxification regime of lofexidine and additional symptomatic medication. He had taken a week off work to do the detoxification, and daily home visits were undertaken.

Lee's progress through the detoxification was uneventful, with poor sleep the most troublesome aspect. He was pleasantly surprised with the low level of withdrawal discomfort, compared to his own attempts to come off heroin without medication. He and his parents followed the instructions carefully, and in all Lee used about three-quarters of the available medication, apart from the sleeping tablets, which were all necessary. Nine days after his last use of heroin naltrexone was instituted, with no withdrawal reaction.

Three months later, Lee remains on naltrexone, and there has been no relapse into heroin use. He is enjoying sporting activities again, and has a holiday abroad planned with some friends. Although he had thought he would still use ecstasy, he appears not to have done so, wanting to try to manage without drugs altogether.

Method 3 – Dihydrocodeine plus symptomatic medication

It has already been indicated in the previous chapter that dihydrocodeine retains its place in the management of opioid dependence, sometimes in maintenance but certainly in detoxification. Perhaps the purist view among specialists would be that where dihydrocodeine was previously used the candidate drug should probably now be buprenorphine, but undoubtedly there are settings where the somewhat more complicated nature of buprenorphine treatment and the higher level of administrative control deter its use. In the literature there is not much to help guide, for instance, police surgeons and others who will use dihydrocodeine as a safe form of detoxification, and so here I have included a description of such use and an example protocol (in the Appendix). Therefore leaving buprenorphine aside until the full discussion later in this chapter, the following still accurately describes a place for dihydrocodeine in our own services.

The medication is typically used for individuals whose heroin usage is not quite heavy enough to justify methadone, but who are considered unlikely to be able to tolerate a fully nonsubstitution method of detoxification. Dihydrocodeine is prescribed according to a fixed regime, which can conclude with the usual combination of outright symptomatic medication, although, importantly, lower levels of these can often be used than in the two previous methods. The dihydrocodeine course can be shortened, as suggested, if the relatively high doses in the first few days are considered unnecessary, or if it is felt there would be a problem in sustaining motivation over the 14-day period. The context of the obvious comparison with buprenorphine has been given, and one disadvantage of the dihydrocodeine method is that any introduction of naltrexone for relapse prevention is more delayed, as a full agonist has been used.

In another example of switching to a different drug to conclude a detoxification, dihydrocodeine itself has been found useful at the tail-end of methadone treatment (Banbery et al. 2000).

Case history

Jane is a 24-year-old single mother with two young children. Following occasional use of other drugs, she was introduced to heroin by her ex-boyfriend. He has had intermittent contact with drug services but proved to be poorly motivated, and he is now serving a prison sentence for supplying drugs. When Jane presented to our service recently she was smoking between 0.5 and 0.75 g of heroin per day, but wanted to stop all drug use and sever her contacts with the drug scene.

Jane had unsuccessfully attempted detoxification with lofexidine about six months previously. At the time she had been keen to have this method and then go on naltrexone, but the main problem had been that she was unable to satisfactorily reduce her heroin use in preparation. She also had the ongoing stresses of child care, although she had had some help offered.

Over the course of two counselling appointments it was clear that Jane would be unable to reduce her heroin substantially before a detoxification, but also that her general motivation was good. The dihydrocodeine method was selected, to give good symptom relief in the early stages of stopping moderate heroin usage. The nature of the treatment was carefully explained and the instructions were made very clear. A friend of Jane's had offered to have her children for much of the time during the detoxification period, and anyway the need for great care in looking after her tablets was emphasized.

At three home visits during the first week it appeared that the detoxification was going according to plan. Jane felt comfortable on the dihydrocodeine until around the start of the second week, when she slightly overused the medication and the stage of symptomatic drugs had to be brought forward. With much support she saw the process through, and managed the nine days from the end of dihydrocodeine which we required before starting naltrexone. In the early stages following detoxification she has experienced some mood disturbance, and she is to be assessed for antidepressant medication.

Clonidine

Clonidine reduces opiate withdrawal symptoms because it acts on the noradrenergic system, and some opiate withdrawal symptoms are due to noradrenergic overactivity. Specifically, it is an alpha-adrenergic agonist which acts preferentially on presynaptic alpha-2 neurons to inhibit noradrenergic transmission, with the action in the locus coeruleus particularly important in relation to opiate use (Gold 1993). The opiate withdrawal symptoms which have a noradrenergic basis include watery eyes, runny nose, sweating, diarrhoea, chills and gooseflesh, and so these are the ones most usually relieved by clonidine and its analogues, lofexidine and guanfacine (San et al. 1990). Clonidine itself, however, has pronounced hypotensive and sedative effects which limit its acceptability and safety in drug misuse treatment. Although in inpatient detoxification with the drug some individuals may actually value the sedation and a related possible anti-anxiety effect, it is usually considered unsuitable for community treatment, when a less toxic analogue can be used.

Methadone

Although in some countries methadone is considered as only suitable for maintenance treatment, in the UK it has also been the mainstay treatment for opiate detoxification. For short-term detoxification its role is currently being reassessed in the light of the use of lofexidine and buprenorphine, and the presentation of many young, early-stage heroin users who do not require or want substitution treatment, but clinics typically also have many individuals on slowly reducing methadone courses. Methadone in general and the role of maintenance treatment were discussed in Chapter 1, while this section examines the subject of detoxification with the drug in some detail, as in services where it is used it is often the main source of problems of practical clinical management. As in the section on maintenance, the observations here which are on outright practicalities increasingly apply to the use of buprenorphine as well, although the separate features of treatment with the latter are considered next.

Suitability as a detoxification medication

Methadone is a hugely useful treatment in drug misuse, including in attempts at withdrawal, but unfortunately its portrayal as a detoxification method usually gives no indication as to how rare uncomplicated completion of treatment actually is. Figure 3.1 is a modified version of the schematic representation of methadone detoxification contained in a previous version of the Department of Health's Guidelines on Clinical Management of Drug Misuse and Dependence (1991) – the representation is the original, while the line indicating problems is my addition, reflecting many other observations such as those by Banbery et al. (2000).

I would contend that in ordinary community treatment of routine cases, the uncomplicated progress of a methadone detoxification by incremental reductions in dose from, say, 35 mg per day, 30, 25…to…10, 5, 4, 3, 2, 1, zero, establishing abstinence as planned at the end, is extremely rare, not to say virtually unknown. In practice many patients manage the first part, but requests will then be made not to reduce, or, if that is not an option, heroin use will re-emerge below a certain threshold dosage. In a medium-dose methadone detoxification, for instance starting at about 50 mg per day, problems will often be encountered at around 15 to 25 mg per day, the issue usually being severity of withdrawal symptoms, which even the best-motivated individuals will find it difficult not to seek to relieve in this relatively slow process. At such a stage decisions need to be taken as to whether to continue with methadone at a stable dosage for a period, whether even to increase to regain the benefits which have been lost, or to switch to one of the previously described methods of quick detoxification.

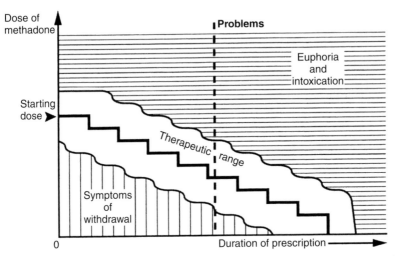

Figure 3.1 The principle of opioid withdrawal by a reducing dose of methadone (adapted from Department of Health, 1991, reproduced with the permission of the Controller of Her Majesty's Stationery Office).

There seems little doubt that it is partly the properties of methadone itself, as well as factors relating to the users, which account for the difficulties seen in detoxification with the drug. The long duration of action and receptor binding properties which contribute to methadone's effectiveness as a stabilizing maintenance medication make it a much less suitable drug for detoxification, and presumably relate to the pervasive and protracted withdrawal symptoms which are frequently experienced. One of the most common observations about methadone is that 'it's worse to come off than heroin', and we should acknowledge that this is almost certainly true (Rosenbaum & Murphy 1984), to be weighed against the undoubted benefits of methadone in many situations. As well as seeing the difficulties of ongoing methadone detoxifications, many clinical workers operate with the assumption that withdrawal symptoms in any detoxification course will be worse if the detoxification is *from methadone*, than if the same course is used *from heroin*. Not many studies directly test this, but Gossop and Strang (1991) found that of heroin and methadone users given a ten-day methadone detoxification, the previous methadone users had more insomnia, muscular tension, weakness and aches and pains, with completion rates similar in an inpatient setting and dosage relatively unimportant. Certainly these symptoms are very familiar as generally the main complaints of individuals coming off methadone, with those who have done so suddenly in prison or residential rehabilitation often reporting that weeks or months have gone by before aching finally goes and sleep returns to normal.

In defence of methadone, the main difficulties some individuals have are of adjusting first to its (relatively) noneuphoriant effect, and then to the prospect of being without drugs altogether (Milby et al. 1986). Methadone is used for more difficult candidates than non-opioid detoxification, and courses may become protracted partly due to actual reluctance to reduce, which compounds any difficulties relating to the drug. If detoxification has been imposed on an individual who is not ready to do it, the particular withdrawal syndrome of methadone is unlikely to be the critical factor, although it may not help.

A methadone detoxification is more often completed if it is done as an inpatient than as an outpatient (Gossop et al. 1986), but many individuals are reluctant to be admitted, and various other limitations of inpatient treatment were indicated in the Introduction. In attempting to provide the most useful combination of treatments in a community setting, we have no problem with offering methadone detoxification as an option, basically in cases where there are not the features favourable for the quicker methods. However, we do not expect it to proceed in a simple manner, and some of the more important practical management considerations are discussed below.

Evidence from studies

Much useful information on methadone detoxification came from a series of studies at the Drug Dependence Unit of the Maudsley Hospital in London in the 1980s. In inpatient treatment, the prolonged opiate withdrawal symptoms in a methadone detoxification were demonstrated, peaking towards the end of the course and lasting at least another 20 days (Gossop et al. 1987). Other inpatient studies found that withdrawal distress is increased if individuals have high levels of anxiety (Phillips et al. 1986), and reduced if detailed information on the nature of withdrawal symptoms is provided (Green & Gossop 1988). A study which found similar levels of withdrawal symptoms in 10- and 21-day methadone courses (Gossop et al. 1989) led to the 10-day course being adopted as standard in that unit, but 10 days would almost always be considered too short for a community detoxification.

In a randomized controlled trial of inpatient and outpatient methadone detoxification (Gossop et al. 1986), completion rates were 81% in inpatients but only 17% (five individuals) in outpatients. Few details of the regimes are given, but the outpatient methadone course lasted eight weeks from an average starting dose of 37.5 mg, and abstinence was apparently confirmed by urinalysis. A study exclusively in outpatients investigated the matter of whether it was preferable to give users a say in their rate of detoxification, as opposed to imposing a fixed regime (Dawe et al. 1991). Users were randomly allocated to either a six-week methadone course which reduced at a set rate, or to a system where they could negotiate their rate of reduction, with the instruction that it was meant to last about the same period. Not surprisingly, only 17% (3) of the flexible group had completed their course by six weeks, the others having not reduced enough or dropped out. Approximately half of each group dropped out, and 40% of all urine samples during detoxification were positive for heroin – similar across the two groups.

Some of the same researchers are still involved in extensive research on methadone, with the UK's most substantial study in recent times being the National Treatment Outcome Research Study (NTORS) (Gossop et al. 2003). This has followed up large cohorts of patients in drug services receiving any of four treatment modalities, with two of these being methadone maintenance and methadone reduction. Outcomes in treatment were measured across many domains, including use of the various types of substances, and mention is made at several points in this book of results for opiate use, alcohol or cocaine use, etc. One of the most striking results regarding the treatment itself showed just how often prescribing called 'reduction' or 'detoxification' in fact becomes ongoing and barely altered: therefore at one year on, patients identified as being in reduction treatment had not lowered their dose significantly more than the patients in methadone maintenance (Gossop et al. 2000), having started at similar levels! Even more damningly, the main drug usage finding in a comparison in an associated paper from the study was that 'the more rapidly the methadone was reduced, the worse the heroin outcomes' (Gossop et al. 2001).

In the light of this it might be thought that any discussion of methadone as an attempted detoxification method could usefully stop here, but a hugely common modern dilemma is whether to actually stand in the way of an individual who overtly states that they wish to reduce their methadone, especially in these days of 'partnerships with patients' and 'patient-centred treatment'. In short, whether rightly or wrongly, currently in UK clinics if patients are adamant that they wish to reduce this medication it will usually be done, which is why the practical problems I have tried to portray and advise on are so common. As an aside, there are indeed various ways in which such a patient-choice agenda could seriously compromise opiate dependence treatment in the future, including whether we accept resistance to giving samples for drug testing, and requests for unsupervised consumption or widely spaced collection of substitute medication which the treating clinician might consider unwise.

Practical issues

Starting dose

Methadone detoxification is nearly always in the form of the 1 mg in 1 ml mixture. Some individuals doing a detoxification from injectable maintenance wish to reduce in that form in the first instance, but clearly a switch to mixture should be made sooner or later, possibly using combinations of the two for a period. Methadone tablets are increasingly discouraged, while the 2 mg in 5 ml linctus may be useful at very low dosages, for ease of measurement.

Conversion tables from street heroin and pharmaceutical opioids are readily available, although these are only a guide, and can sometimes be quite an unreliable one, for instance because of different half-lives and the non-linear equivalence relationships between drugs. At one time there was the rather convenient situation in the UK whereby pounds in money of street heroin could be used as a rough guide to mg requirement in methadone, but now there are great variations in street heroin purity, and tighter recommendations for a starting methadone dose – often to be 40 mg per day, according to the Department of Health (2007). Any conversions of course follow assessment of quality of information and confirmation of history, including testing. Admission to hospital for titration of dosage against withdrawal signs used to be fairly routine, but a titration approach is usually now considered impracticable in community treatment, if only because of numbers presenting. It is therefore necessary to be conservative in terms of the starting dosage, and this can be reviewed in the light of any remaining withdrawal effects at subsequent appointments. The unusual and highly dangerous property of methadone should be borne in mind, that a dose that is correct for an individual for whom methadone is indicated is readily fatal to any non-tolerant person, with lowering of that threshold if additional drugs are taken. Increasingly, supervised consumption of methadone can be at a user's local community pharmacy premises rather than requiring a trip to the treatment centre, which makes daily dispensing even more routine. For those who have had methadone unofficially in the street scene, it is useful to explain that the dose required in guaranteed daily treatment is less than they may have taken in an 'emergency' when withdrawing from heroin, in more erratic usage.

Individuals who have been misusing pharmaceutical opioids pose a particular problem, as any straight conversion from claimed average usage tends to result in methadone dosages which appear excessively high. In practice, such users can usually be given doses of methadone typical of routine treatment, as good progress is often made once the supportive elements of management are also in place.

Even in a short-term detoxification, an initial stabilizing period on the same methadone dose is often desirable, so that the user gains confidence in the treatment, and the effects of cessation of other drugs can be gauged before dose reduction. Further counselling on the withdrawal process can be done in this period, as typically some aspects do not 'sink in' while negotiation to secure methadone treatment is still under way.

Dispensing intervals

Although some users may be reluctant to agree to daily dispensing, it is difficult to argue a good case against it in the initial stages, when it is so important that the correct daily dosage is guaranteed. If it is unpopular, the matter of dispensing intervals can be used in the standard kind of behavioural approach, where there is some relaxation of the arrangement if good progress is shown. We prefer to revert to daily dispensing at the end of a detoxification, however, when small amounts are involved and stability is vital.

Contracts

The more that treatment with methadone and buprenorphine has moved towards 'harm-reduction' policies, the rarer set treatment contracts have become. Services may have a document for patients to sign regarding clinic systems, such as requirements in attending appointments and behaviours which are prohibited in the building, but formal contracts indicating sanctions for additional drug use or other forms of poor compliance are unusual. Such issues have been discussed in relation to maintenance treatment, while in detoxification it may be more advisable to lay down the requirements and implications in treatment somewhat more systematically, for instance the rate of reduction of medication (see below). Indeed the prime place for such specifics is with medications for which there is no consensus supporting ongoing prescribing, particularly benzodiazepines, rather than in the main methadone or buprenorphine treatment, for which a halt in reduction could almost always be justified by evidence from studies.

Rate of reduction

The practice of having an initial stabilizing period on the selected starting dose of methadone has been referred to, as has the strong likelihood of encountering problems with withdrawal symptoms towards the end of a detoxification. We expect to change to another form of treatment when the methadone dose is down to about 10–20mg per day, and we broadly acknowledge this with the patient, although attempting to avoid actually inducing problems through suggestion. Between these stages, there is simply not enough evidence relating to community (as opposed to inpatient) treatment to recommend any set period for a methadone detoxification, or therefore any particular rate of reduction. If it is unlikely anyway that a detoxification will be continued to its conclusion, the findings of Dawe et al. (1991), referred to above, are not strong enough to definitely favour a fixed rather than a flexible schedule, and we offer users a say in the rate at which they will reduce. If the starting dose is, say, 40mg per day, it might be proposed to reduce the daily dose by 5mg each two weeks, or each four weeks, and it is useful to do the arithmetic with the patient and calculate how long a detoxification would take at that rate. The longer courses merge into the model of what is often called slow outpatient detoxification, as if that is inherently a more comfortable approach.

Psychologically, some individuals who are motivated to detoxify nevertheless do not like to see their daily dose of methadone visibly reduce, claiming that this produces further anxiety, and for them we can provide a 'fixed volume reduction'. In this approach the volume of liquid remains the same while the methadone constituent gradually decreases, or to avoid excessive dilution at very low methadone dosages the volume may also reduce, but to a lesser extent. We adopt this method only when a patient has requested it, but by definition once the process is under way they are unaware of their exact methadone dosage, the pharmacist being requested not to divulge the information. In our experience this approach probably does not increase the rate of straightforward completion of methadone detoxification, but it can be effective in enabling substantial reductions in dosage in some cases.

Additional medication

It is preferable to use additional symptomatic medication only for specific opiate with-drawal symptoms, anxiety or insomnia when a switch is made from methadone reduction to another detoxification package (see below). The aspect of additional benzodiazepine use by methadone patients has been considered in Chapter 2, and can pose major practical problems in methadone detoxification. If benzodiazepines have been established alongside methadone maintenance treatment, then when the time comes for any requested metha-done reduction there is often a temptation for individuals to at least want to continue the benzodiazepines, if not increase them to compensate for the reduction in methadone – in other words, as we frequently point out to patients in clinic, just the 'wrong way round' in terms of approval for ongoing treatment. Clearly, even if a methadone detoxification is successful there may then be an established high-dose benzodiazepine dependence to address, and the reality may be a confused situation somewhere in between. In short-term methadone detoxification, the temptation to add benzodiazepines for insomnia at an early stage should be resisted, as tolerance to the hypnotic effect of benzodiazepines occurs relatively quickly, and so by the time a user really needs them, at the very end of a detoxification, they may have lost their effectiveness. Increasingly alternatives to benzodi-azepines are used such as zopiclone or zolpidem, as discussed in Chapter 2, but overall it is fanciful to think that outpatient methadone withdrawal will often take place without a perceived need for sleeping tablets, with detoxification using methadone particularly problematic in this way (Beswick et al. 2003).

In addition to its use as a primary detoxification agent, lofexidine is used by some clinicians as an adjunctive treatment in a methadone detoxification, to help reduce the ongoing symptoms as reduction occurs. This is not the recommended usage, and a con-trolled study found guanfacine ineffective in this regard (San et al. 1994).

Another complication which can be expected in a methadone detoxification, seemingly more even than in other methods, is that of mood disturbances. In a comparison of methadone and buprenorphine withdrawal courses, actually in addition to carbamazepine, Seifert et al. (2005) found more tiredness, sensitivity in mood and depression in the (randomly assigned) methadone patients, which situation can lead to either tranquillizers or antidepressants being considered.

Partial detoxifications

If the difficulties encountered in a methadone detoxification are largely due to inability to tolerate the withdrawal features, the problems often start somewhere between one-half and three-quarters of the way through a planned reduction course. Problems much before this perhaps suggest other factors relating more to the individual, and in all cases when problems occur there must be a reappraisal of a patient's circumstances and of their prospects for detoxification. Sometimes it will appear that detoxification is too ambitious an aim, and that the individual may require long-term treatment. In other cases detoxification may still be desired, but an individual's personal or social situation may be conspiring against a successful outcome. Often a series of counselling sessions with a drug worker is required to make suitable plans, and the methadone dose may be held at the same level for a limited period while this is done. If a detoxification is to continue but definite problems with the reduction are being encountered, it is nearly always preferable to switch to one of the other withdrawal methods outlined in this chapter, if necessary with some modifications.

With the availability of methadone, buprenorphine and lofexidine, plus symptomatic medication only and inpatient and even experimental methods, many switches of treatment are possible, and several of these have been discussed, such as going from methadone to buprenorphine (Glasper et al. 2005) and methadone to dihydrocodeine (Banbery et al. 2000). Another modern feature is the lack of any insistence on full detoxification at any stage, and so a wide variety of daily dosages are encountered in practice, any of which may represent partial reductions. Such a situation, when a patient may have come down from for instance 80 mg to 60 mg per day and then remained there, can be satisfactory, and often is viewed as progress by patients. Clearly clinicians must always see that there has not been some compensatory drawback, such as relapse into more drug use or an increase in drinking. We should not perhaps always be nervous of patients' wishes to reduce, taking into consideration that the studies with extremely poor results from detoxification have often been when that condition was enforced. There are a few papers in the literature which specifically examine slow methadone reductions in clinics which also encourage indefinite maintenance, although even then results of reduction attempts are not what could be called good. Calsyn et al. (2006) found that in a programme which 'support(ed) both tapering attempts and indefinite maintenance' the commonest reasons for patients halting their reductions were feeling unstable, including with mood disturbances, and return of drug use, with needing relief of pain also mentioned.

Topic in brief – 8. Methadone detoxification

- Undoubtedly leads to more relapsing into substance abuse and associated problems than methadone maintenance
- Is nevertheless carried out if requested by users within 'patient-centred' policies
- Appears even more uncomfortable than other detoxifications in mood disturbances, sleep problems, pain symptoms and general distress
- If from maintenance methadone with associated benzodiazepine prescribing, often involves requests for continued or increased benzodiazepines and therefore 'wrong way round' treatment

---

Buprenorphine

The profile of buprenorphine has been discussed in Chapter 2, a partial opioid agonist and partial antagonist with several potential advantages as a direct alternative to methadone. The prominence which the medication has reached within treatment, actually in about the time since the first edition of this book, has also been referred to at several points, and as well as appearing broadly equivalent in effectiveness to methadone for maintenance, it has even more appeal as a detoxification option. This is mainly because of the evidence suggesting significantly less severe withdrawal symptoms than methadone, both in terms of the symptoms which emerge when it is used rather than methadone as a detoxification from heroin, but also regarding the severity when the two medications are compared in reducing from maintenance treatment. The second advantage in detoxification is that the opiate antagonist naltrexone can be started as little as one to two days after the last dose of buprenorphine (Rosen & Kosten 1995), whereas if methadone has been the detoxification medication the wait is more like 7–10 days.

The literature on buprenorphine is now substantial, and this section will refer to a fairly representative sample of studies which illustrate points that are important for practice. The relatively mild nature of the abstinence syndrome has been demonstrated in animal and human studies, even when withdrawal is precipitated by opiate antagonists (Negus & Woods 1995). Perhaps because it has been recognized for decades that methadone's features make that seemingly much more suitable as a maintenance than detoxification medication, most of the comparative studies of buprenorphine in detoxification following its introduction were against symptomatic agents such as clonidine. In these comparisons buprenorphine was found to provide clearly better symptom relief (Gowing et al. 2004), with the randomized controlled trial of buprenorphine against clonidine by Lintzeris et al. (2002) specifically demonstrating superiority of buprenorphine in better retention during and even after treatment, less heroin use and less withdrawal comfort. The main author also provided an example of a reducing buprenorphine protocol over just eight days which proved mainly satisfactory in a small trial, with mild withdrawal severity and minimal rebound on cessation of dosing (Lintzeris 2002). Even during the course of that exploratory investigation there was an alteration from early subjects receiving just 4mg on day one to later subjects receiving 6 or 8mg, because of inadequate initial symptom relief, and the latter reflects dosing very commonly used in practice currently. In that systematic protocol doses for days two and three were 8 to 12mg, and this is certainly very similar to what we do in our own outpatients, with, however, then a reduction course which can last more like 2–3 weeks.

As mentioned earlier in the chapter, in the UK lofexidine is far more frequently selected in opiate detoxification than clonidine because of its better safety for outpatients, and a large comparative study of this and buprenorphine was carried out by Raistrick et al. (2005). Two hundred and ten patients were randomized, and the same comparisons in standard drug misuse outcomes and satisfaction measures were also studied in 271 individuals who did not wish to be in the randomized study. Many outcomes were similar with the two medications, but 65% of buprenorphine patients completed detoxification against 46% of those on lofexidine. That study was an example of one which included a follow-up to see whether patients had been abstinent after detoxification, with this being the case at the measurement point of one month for 38% of lofexidine completers and 46% with buprenorphine. This important aspect of whether 'successful' detoxification does indeed lead to further abstinence has attracted attention in several buprenorphine studies, as reviewed by Horspool et al. (2008). Across five qualifying studies, they found detoxification completion rates of 65 to 100%, but low rates of abstinence at follow-up points, with more patients having returned to opioid maintenance than had complied with naltrexone.

A one-month follow-up was included in a study by Breen et al. (2003) which used buprenorphine for detoxification as a transfer from methadone, with a 31% abstinence rate at that point. This investigation was also of interest as an illustration of much longer detoxification courses, in which patients had some choice in their reduction rate: individuals who transferred from a methadone dose of 30 mg took an average of 12.5 weeks to reduce to zero buprenorphine if they did indeed complete, while if the transfer was below 30 mg of methadone the reduction to zero buprenorphine took on average 8.3 weeks.

Whatever the length of detoxification, the issue of some symptomatic medication such as hypnotics at the very end can arise just as with methadone or dihydrocodeine, but there has been no informative investigation of this aspect.

Inpatient treatment

The general issues concerning inpatient treatment of drug misusers have been discussed in the Introduction, and the use of methadone and buprenorphine detoxification treatments in this chapter. Many of the problems of methadone detoxification, including the risks of misuse and diversion, and noncompletion due to inability to tolerate the prolonged withdrawal effects, are reduced in inpatient treatment, and use of the drug remains a valid approach in that setting, with the various provisos referred to above. However, the methadone courses may last three weeks or even more and, with length of stay identified as an important issue by both patients and treatment providers, there is currently much interest in regimes which can achieve detoxification from opiates more quickly.

As indicated, buprenorphine can offer a quicker option than methadone, with a three-day course reported to be effective for withdrawal from heroin (Cheskin et al. 1994). The side-effects of clonidine which render it unsuitable for community treatment can be manageable in the inpatient setting, although the drug is being superseded by lofexidine where that is available. Controlled studies have found clonidine and lofexidine to be equally effective in alleviating withdrawal symptoms in inpatient detoxification from heroin (Lin et al. 1997) and from methadone (Khan et al. 1997), with lofexidine resulting in less hypotension and fewer adverse effects. Another double-blind controlled study found lofexidine to be broadly as effective as a ten-day methadone detoxification in inpatient opiate withdrawal (Bearn et al. 1996).

The terms 'rapid opioid detoxification' and 'accelerated withdrawal' are used to refer to techniques in which withdrawal is actually precipitated by administration of an opiate antagonist, and then non-opiate drugs are used to manage the symptoms. Various regimes have been described, using either naltrexone or intravenous naloxone at the outset, and clonidine, lofexidine and sedatives (e.g. Merrill & Marshall 1997, Beaini et al. 2000). The most severe techniques are carried out under heavy sedation or even general anaesthesia (Tretter et al. 1998, Kaye et al. 2003, Krabbe et al. 2003). Rapid detoxification, particularly under anaesthesia, has received a good deal of publicity, and can catch the imagination of older users in particular who still retain a desire to detoxify, but have become disillusioned with conventional, longer methods. A distinction seems to be often drawn between the relatively well-tried methods virtually confined to naltrexone and clonidine or lofexidine, and the more severe experimental techniques. For instance, in a brief report, Rumball and Williams (1997) made claims for their routine method over eight years' experience, and considered that, by contrast, 'it is the introduction of anaesthesia and polypharmacy to the process that has...quite unnecessarily introduced major hazards'. They reported high acceptability, provided patients were excluded who may also be withdrawing from benzodiazepines or alcohol, had used large or unquantifiable amounts of opiates, or had serious physical illness or lack of venous access. The basic rapid detoxification techniques have indeed become widespread, partly through a desire to make more efficient use of inpatient units. It should at least prove possible to reduce the proportion of individuals who fail to complete a detoxification, if only because the period involved is shorter.

It is, however, detoxification under general anaesthesia which has attracted the most publicity in the media, and perhaps the most interest on the part of community patients. It is often alleged by drug misuse specialists that a condition which is not itself dangerous, opiate withdrawal, does not justify the risks of an anaesthetic. However, proponents of the method point out that the same argument is not always used in, say, childbirth or dental treatment, and there is a case for weighing the risks of anaesthetic against not only those of withdrawal, but also those of ongoing drug misuse. That case would be stronger if it were shown that detoxification under anaesthetic led to higher abstinence rates than other methods, but only a few direct comparisons are available (e.g. Krabbe et al. 2003).

There is clearly further debate among those who carry out the different ultra-rapid experimental techniques as to whether the risks of an anaesthetic, in a relatively young person without any invasive procedure being performed, are actually greater than those where very high doses of oral sedatives are managed by a psychiatrist, with no conclusion on that really possible.

Relapse prevention

Naltrexone

Naltrexone is a long-acting competitive opiate antagonist which is effective orally (Gonzalez & Brogden 1988). It can be used to precipitate withdrawal in accelerated detoxification from opiates (see above), but its main use in community treatment is as a relapse-prevention strategy (Farren 1997). The principle of treatment is that on establishing a dosage of one 50 mg tablet per day, any ordinary amounts of opiates which are subsequently taken are rendered completely ineffective, the medication therefore acting as a strong disincentive to drug use. This resembles the use of disulfiram in alcohol abuse, but with the great advantage that there is no dangerous interaction to guard against, and so it can be used much more freely. In our regimes for quick detoxification from heroin which I have described above, naltrexone is an integral part of the treatment package, which users are briefed about from the start. Indeed, given the general difficulty of staying off heroin in communities where it is freely available, we find individuals presenting whose main motivation is to have treatment with 'the blockers'. In turn, one of our reasons for often selecting lofexidine as a detoxification method is that naltrexone can be established straightaway on completion of the withdrawal course, since an opioid has not been used, and even the partial agonist buprenorphine enables the gap period to be much shorter than it is with methadone. This combination of detoxification then naltrexone is often attempted in UK services, but we feel that to be successful with this type of user naltrexone must be assertively encouraged from the outset. Our view – and apparently that of the users – is that relapse rates in opiate misuse are such that there needs to be a good reason *not* to include this relatively straightforward treatment option, for a period, in attempting to enhance an individual's chances of success.

Regarding effectiveness of naltrexone, it has never ceased to amaze me how naltrexone tends to be portrayed in the literature, almost as if it is some kind of direct alternative to methadone in the same indications. If very recently active long-standing opiate addicts are given methadone or naltrexone, the finding that retention and avoidance of drugs are higher with 'agonist than antagonist maintenance' is completely unsurprising, and it should simply be recognized that naltrexone is an option for people at a particular stage of treatment, i.e. after elective withdrawal. I remember making a similar point at a meeting of specialists from various countries once, i.e. querying the sense of doing comparisons in active users, and an eminent specialist in international psychiatry explained that part of the reason they were done was to persuade countries that do not have methadone to introduce it. Perhaps it is a reflection of the slightly peculiar status of naltrexone within treatment that, many years later, I have never quite worked out whether I find that motive somewhat justifiable, or absolutely outrageous!

Certainly here I will not reproduce the efforts of systematic reviews, which cover a wide range of studies including those with the issue mentioned above and have mainly been pessimistic about naltrexone. Also I will not go down the route of concentrating on special groups such as those on court orders or addicted professionals, although it is easy to see why if much is at stake – an avoidance of return to custody, or a career – such individuals may make better than average progress (Ward et al. 1999). Clearly naltrexone can be extremely useful in a proportion of patients, and indeed given that the standard dose produces complete blockade it unquestionably 'works' at one level provided it is actually taken. Stopping taking the tablets is the usual precursor to a relapse into opiate abuse, with Bartu et al. (2002) finding individuals often then re-presenting for further treatment, on average after intervals of three to four months. A meta-analysis by Johansson et al. (2006) examined 15 studies involving 1071 patients, with full outcome measures available in ten studies, and found retention in treatment to be the strongest influence on efficacy, but that anyway naltrexone was significantly better than non-substitution treatment control conditions in objective demonstrations of abstinence. They showed that the results of naltrexone treatment tended to be improved by the addition of contingency management, i.e. providing rewards for abstinence, echoing the findings in another demanding area discussed in the next chapter, the management of cocaine abuse. Other behaviour therapies and even antidepressants have sometimes been found to be useful, and in a study of 72 patients by Stella et al. (1999), higher drug-free rates occurred when additional psychological support, testing and involvement of staff in supervising naltrexone were in place. A further point on the interpretation of studies and reputation of naltrexone is that the definition of 'failure' is, inevitably but paradoxically, harsher in studies of antagonist than substitution treatments: that is, any relapse into opiate use will be classed as a naltrexone failure, whereas studies of methadone will claim success even when reduced amounts of substances are taken in addition to the substitute opioid (see Hulse & Basso, 1999, for an analysis relating to this).

A few practical aspects will now be discussed. The tablets may be crushed up in a liquid, preferably something like a fruit juice as there is a bitter taste. No depot preparation is very widely used, but the issue is briefly indicated below. Naltrexone should probably not be used in those with significantly impaired liver function, as abnormal liver function tests have been demonstrated in treatment with a much higher dose, used for obesity. Side-effects at the 50mg dose may include headaches, dizziness, nausea and feelings which resemble mild withdrawal such as chills or abdominal discomfort. Various mood disturbances are common in the early stages of treatment, but these may often be related to the absence of mood-altering drugs and the general process of adjustment, producing for instance some frustration or irritability. From a comparison of pharmacological and clinical data in alcohol, opioid and nicotine studies, Miotto et al. (2002) felt that the dysphoria which commonly occurs after withdrawal did not in the opioid cases seem to be attributable to the naltrexone.

Because of the nature of naltrexone treatment it is clearly necessary to have been opiate-free for a period before starting, with the length of this depending on the treatment drug, as already described. If a non-opioid method of detoxification is employed, the days actually in this treatment can of course be included if no opiate use has occurred. The manufacturers of naltrexone have recommended that a challenge with intravenous naloxone is performed to detect, by the presence or absence of precipitated withdrawal symptoms, whether the period off opiates has been adequate. Increasingly, however, services are using a small dose of oral naltrexone itself for this purpose. In common with others, we find that in detoxification from small amounts of heroin the opiate-free period does not need to be as long as seven days, and that naltrexone can often be introduced cautiously from about four days onwards. Our users are often impatient to start, and indeed derive a strong psychological advantage from doing so, and treatment can be initiated at a quarter of a tablet for a day or so, moving to half a tablet and then the full one tablet per day by the standard 7–10 day opiate-free stage. Supervision of the first dose by the worker is desirable, with 30–60 minutes' observation for withdrawal symptoms.

There is little evidence to bring to bear on the question of how long naltrexone treatment should continue. Several studies have used a six-month period, including one which found no advantage of naltrexone over placebo, notably in polydrug users with lengthy histories (San et al. 1991). As with disulfiram, there is probably no set period which is preferable, with much individual variation in availability of supervision, extent of exposure to risky situations, motivating factors and toleration of the drug. We routinely use naltrexone for four weeks in the initial period of adjustment after detoxification, and then recommend continuation for three to six months if there are no problems of acceptability. It is not uncommon for users to test out naltrexone by having an amount of heroin, and, although any drug use in such circumstances is unfortunate, at least it is then recognized that the blockade does indeed work. 'Over-riding' the effects of naltrexone probably requires taking four or five times an average heroin dose, and is not attempted in the population in which we are using the medication.

It is possible to have various reservations about naltrexone treatment, and there are clear limitations as well as some potential for what may be broadly termed misuse. Brewer (1996) criticized the ideological objection to naltrexone, from those who believe that motivation to abstain from drugs can only truly come from an individual's personal psychological resources. Recognition of relapse rates is probably sufficient for most clinicians to avoid adhering to that position rigidly, but the view is encountered in some settings which practise particular purist treatment models, such as some residential rehabilitation centres. More in terms of general clinical impressions, some workers feel that naltrexone probably works best in those who would have managed well without it anyway, but this has not really been tested and is not in itself an objection to the treatment. A definite limitation of the treatment is that it clearly only acts in relation to opiates, and so cannot prevent relapse into other drug misuse.

In using naltrexone treatment widely, we have occasionally encountered various inappropriate usages of the medication. One type of situation extends out of the proper use, but without full compliance of the patient. Thus, a relative or partner may insist on naltrexone being continued even when they suspect that relapse has taken place, or alternatively they may resort to concealed administration. One woman who was exasperated by her partner's failure to take the medication put it in his cup of tea, but unfortunately their friend who was an active user drank this by mistake, and promptly became very ill with withdrawal symptoms. Some parents have realized that giving naltrexone can test whether their child is on heroin, and one teenager presented to us in severe withdrawal having had this done. Drink-'spiking' with naltrexone is also emerging, seemingly done to users by their friends for amusement purposes. Users themselves may misguidedly decide to take naltrexone to attempt a quick self-detoxification, which is a potentially dangerous situation, particularly in impulsive heavily dependent polydrug users. All these inappropriate uses have implications for the security of naltrexone treatment, which requires a good degree of reliability on the part of patients and their associates who will supervise the treatment, or otherwise controlled dispensing conditions. Our experience has mainly been with well-motivated early-stage heroin users, very different from the forensic or professional groups with whom naltrexone has sometimes previously been associated, and in general we find very high levels of acceptability and a low rate of treatment-related problems.

Only brief mention will be made of the implant or depot preparations of naltrexone, as they are not established in the kind of community services described in this book. Indeed in Sheffield we have conspicuously avoided this option, as a nearby project using it has attracted much controversy, although the treatment is still available to our local addicts. In clinical terms, the very obvious risk is that a user may be put forward for the long-acting implant, perhaps by desperate relatives, but if the individual is not themselves inclined to stay off drugs the potential for relapse into other types, such as cocaine, benzodiazepines or alcohol, is huge. It is not just in our area that the method is controversial, with much debate surrounding projects which offer this treatment in various parts of the world, and it seems that particular problems do arise if there is over-enthusiasm for this one approach, rather than offering naltrexone to people who are suited to it. A good account of treatment with subcutaneous naltrexone implants has been given by Carreno et al. (2003), with definitely impressive results in a clinic with much experience in the treatment.

Case history

Kerry had a one-year history of heroin use before undergoing a straightforward community detoxification with lofexidine and symptomatic medication. She was keen to go on naltrexone, and we supervised the first half-tablet dose, eight days after her last use of heroin. Her mother had helped her through the detoxification at home, and was also going to make sure that Kerry had her naltrexone each day. They were given a patient information leaflet, and a medical warning card for Kerry to carry with her at all times.

Taking naltrexone posed no problems, with her mother good at remembering and, particularly in the early stages, checking to see that Kerry had not secreted the tablet in her mouth. They had a good relationship and Kerry had no objection to the situation being managed in this way. She initially experienced some headaches, but after a week on the medication these went away.

Kerry was regularly seen by her drug worker during treatment with naltrexone. She checked whether she could use cannabis and alcohol while on the medication, and did continue to use these intermittently. On one occasion only, she 'tested out' the naltrexone by using heroin, but reported that she had no effect from the drug. She also said that

Table 3.2 Areas to cover in relapse prevention counselling

Tactics in avoiding active drug users
Dealing with craving and trigger situations
Making realistic short-term plans
Time management
Reinforce need for complete abstinence from drug

she generally did not crave heroin, and clearly saw this as a consequence of being on naltrexone – 'because you know you can't have it, you don't wind yourself up thinking about it'.

After four months Kerry considered that she was at very little risk of using heroin again, and did not want to take the naltrexone any more. She felt that taking the tablet was itself an unnecessary reminder of heroin, which she would manage to avoid because she was determined not to go back to that previous lifestyle. Her mother was nervous about this change, but at subsequent monthly appointments, which Kerry had still requested, there has been no evidence of relapse.

General methods

Not all those who have stopped taking opiates, or drugs in general, require counselling in relapse prevention. It has been observed that cigarette smokers who give up mainly get on with consolidating abstinence themselves, and do not have sessions discussing personal issues. Certainly it can be a mistake to bring recently detoxified drug users back to a busy clinic, where they will find the waiting-room conversations about drugs distressing, and there may be attempts by others to undermine their abstinence. However, we find that many users who have had contact and support through a community detoxification do want to continue seeing their worker for a period afterwards, when various difficulties may be encountered. We offer this in the form of home visits, to ensure contact and also because group meetings can be too risky in the early stages. We favour relapse prevention groups for alcohol misusers, but with drugs there is probably a higher risk that one individual who has relapsed will 'bring the others down', for instance by bringing drugs in. Where an individual does request ongoing visits and counselling, we do this for as long as it appears useful at increasingly spaced appointments, often tied in with naltrexone treatment.

The principles of relapse prevention counselling are similar across the range of drugs, the main theoretical influences being the work of Marlatt & Gordon (1985) and the technique of motivational interviewing (Noonan & Moyers 1997). Drug workers of all disciplines carry out such counselling, and a practical guide from the nursing perspective has been provided by Salazar (1997).

A wide range of adjustments need to be made after detoxification, in many different individual circumstances. Long-term maintenance patients who detoxify may have few or no peers who are not drug users and little remaining from a drug-free lifestyle, with therefore much rebuilding to do. Younger heroin users who go through a quick detoxification, as described at the start of this chapter, usually have a more intact social situation but have to make their adjustments to being abstinent in a very short period. Overall, the practical issues which our team workers find most important to address after detoxification are indicated in Table 3.2.

Avoiding acquaintances who are still using drugs is usually crucial, however solitary it renders an individual's situation (hopefully temporarily). Other users may be envious and attempt to continue contact as if nothing had happened, and dealers do not take kindly to losing a regular customer. Families and partners can be involved in rejecting such approaches, and the worker can help advise on the tactics required. One of our clients wrote to us about the difficulties of separating from other users after detoxification:

You are probably aware that the heroin culture that is quickly emerging, is based on a sense of kinship, a need to belong to an identifiable group. While in this group, young people find that sense of belonging that is missing, whether due to unemployment, or other problems. Subsequently the descent into a habit they simply cannot afford to sustain by normal means is swift. The route out of the habit is not so easy, largely because of the fact that ex-users are subsequently shunned by their peers. I would go as far as to draw the analogy that going 'clean' is tantamount to one of a group of burglars suddenly joining the Police. This in turn regenerates the feeling of isolation that being a user suppresses, and so it is easier to stay on the stuff than to be subjected to the stigma of coming off.

Craving can be problematic, as can trigger situations, usually localities or having money. The day on which a benefit payment or wage is received is especially difficult if money has previously translated into drugs, and tactics are required to spend it on necessities or other things that are desired. Dealing with craving usually involves various methods of distraction, suitable for each individual. Planning new activities is important, but this must be realistic and involve definite action in the short term. Thus if going to college is planned, this involves obtaining information, making decisions about courses and submitting applications at organized times, with guidance. There is usually a vacuum of time to fill in the initial stages, in contrast to previous involvement in raising money and using drugs, and time management advice is useful. Also some 'myths' about drug use can require de-bunking, particularly where individuals feel they could safely use their drug occasionally on a 'treat' basis – the impossibility of doing this with heroin in particular often needs stressing.

Boredom is a great enemy in this situation, with marked differences between areas and countries in the likelihood of gaining employment. In our areas unemployment generally is at high levels, and drug users can feel as if they have few or no prospects. There is no establishment of special schemes whereby users who have detoxified can secure employment as part of rehabilitation, and we often have to provide much encouragement and practical help to seek the few opportunities that there are. The probation service can sometimes offer places on schemes for ex-offenders in particular.

The biggest single adjustment which has to be made on detoxification is that to being without the effects of a mood-altering drug. Clearly, some revert to heroin because of an inability to make this adjustment, but others will switch to a different drug, perhaps one they used earlier in their 'career', or commonly alcohol if they have determined to try to do without drugs. Alcohol is in some ways a particular risk, as those wishing to separate from the drug scene can aim to reintegrate with their previous friends who 'just go out drinking'. Where alcohol use does become excessive shortly after giving up opiates we often find this to be a phase which subsides, but there can come a point where alcohol or any other drug misuse becomes problematic enough to require treatment in its own right or, where relevant, to raise the possibility of reestablishing previous maintenance methadone. The study by Eklund et al. (1994) which illustrates this phenomenon in relation to detoxification from methadone was discussed on page 16.

Other observations

Clinical psychologists are not very numerous in community drug services in the UK and, as already noted, counselling techniques originally derived from this discipline are usually carried out by other workers. Something of a balance needs to be struck here: psychological and behavioural methods are most purely administered by clinical psychologists, but counselling clearly needs to be more widely available, and drug users can be scathing of therapists in generic services who 'don't know anything about drugs', typically failing to comply if they think that the case. We would tend to look to input from specialists, preferably within a drug service but if necessary from elsewhere, in cases where risk of relapse appears to be related to long-standing problems of a psychological nature. Some drug users undoubtedly appear to 'self-medicate' to relieve distress from painful previous experiences, of which child sexual abuse is prominent, and this phenomenon needs addressing if abstinence from drugs is attempted. Where family dynamics appear an important causal or perpetuating factor in an individual's drug misuse, systematic family therapy is another area which requires specialist handling.

Many drug misusers derive benefit from the Narcotics Anonymous organization, whose methods are well known and importantly include an unequivocal commitment to total abstinence from all substances, regular attendance at meetings, and a fellowship of ex-users who can be contacted for support (Gossop et al. 2008). Our own experience is that this approach finds favour with only a relatively small minority of the users who attend clinical services, noticeably smaller than the proportion of alcohol misusers who respond to the generally better-established Alcoholics Anonymous. Probably subcultural differences between the two groups are important, while also our young drug users typically cannot comprehend a future without social use of alcohol, risky though this is.

Treatment
Treatment of non-opiate misuse

Introduction

This book is mainly concerned with the treatment of opiate misuse, for the simple reason that that is the form of drug misuse for which there are the most effective clinical approaches. As we have discussed, the treatment scene for opiate misusers, in contrast to other groups, is fundamentally altered by the widespread availability of the substitution option, in the form of methadone or alternative opioids. Physical dependence is part of the rationale for that approach, and the occurrence of clear-cut withdrawal symptoms also indicates the use of drugs such as lofexidine or clonidine, followed where possible by naltrexone. For reasons of severity of dependence and treatment options, it is therefore understandable that services are inclined to have caseloads dominated by opiate users.

This does not mean that there is nothing that can be done for other drug misusers, although that is the message which is sometimes conveyed. In the UK when the major expansion of methadone services occurred from the 1980s, there was a definite impression of helplessness regarding managing users of non-opiate drugs. Low-threshold prescribing had been advocated for opiate addicts at that time of high perceived HIV threat, partly for engagement purposes, and the community drug services were encouraged to prioritize such treatment, with counselling approaches becoming neglected. If amphetamine users or other groups presented, the often openly asked question was 'if we can't prescribe, what can we do with them?', and the same difficulty can be expressed now by primary care providers trained mainly in the methadone response. As indicated elsewhere, the prescribing ethos has led to experimentation with that approach for some stimulant users, but in a further process of development general counselling skills are requiring rediscovery, ironically partly due to the numbers of newly dependent low-level heroin users presenting and not solely requiring methadone maintenance. Clearly the range of counselling skills and specific behavioural methods are even more necessary in the treatment of non-opiate misuse, where there are precious few effective pharmacological treatments.

General counselling for drug misusers is discussed in Chapter 5, and the particular methods in situations of detoxification and relapse prevention in Chapter 3. The more expertly a service can provide counselling methods, the more confident it can be in managing non-opiate misusers, and possibly even attracting such groups. This is increasingly necessary at the present time given the rise particularly in cocaine abuse, while there has always been an important potential preventive role in intervening in the forms of drug use which are often direct precursors to starting heroin. This chapter will therefore examine the main clinical treatment options for each form of non-opiate drug misuse in turn.

Table 4.1 Important features of cocaine misuse

Rise of 'crack' form, more addictive
Minority of users develop extreme usage
Often periodic
More medically dangerous than heroin
Psychotic features common
Various links with violent crime

Cocaine

Most of our knowledge of treating cocaine misuse comes from the USA, initially following the massive epidemic of the problem there throughout the 1980s (Withers et al. 1995). In the middle of that decade it was estimated that approximately one-tenth of the population had used cocaine, and while no other country has had an equivalent experience, severe cocaine-related problems are encountered in many areas, including the UK's major cities. This is especially so where cocaine is substantially used in the 'crack' form, which is associated with generally higher levels of the various adverse effects and social complications. Some of the important features of cocaine misuse are indicated in Table 4.1.

The transition from cocaine hydrochloride to crack has greatly changed this drug usage. Claims used to be made for the hydrochloride as a harmless desirable accompaniment to the executive lifestyle and, apart from the well-known complication of damage to the nasal septum from snorting, millions of individuals no doubt have used cocaine powder with relatively few adverse effects. (The injected use by polydrug users, for instance in combination with heroin, is inherently much more hazardous.) Crack is produced from cocaine hydrochloride by a simple chemical process, and this purer, more volatile form is much more potent in both effects and withdrawal symptoms. Very rapid rises in blood levels of the drug are achieved by smoking, and this method, using various forms of apparatus, is the main route of administration, although habitual drug injectors will break crack down and inject it. Crack can be said to be more addictive, if that term is used to include the profound psychological features which occur rather than bodily withdrawal symptoms. In particular, craving and acute depressive feelings on withdrawal can be extremely severe, and partly account for the rapidly escalating usage of a minority of individuals. The extent to which individuals become 'hooked' in such ways is very variable with crack, and so while many appear to take the drug on an occasional basis without problems, others develop a compulsive, and indeed extreme, form of usage, spending vast amounts of money in short spaces of time. Fortunately such a pattern is not usually sustainable, although recent research has shown a higher proportion of individuals to maintain similar heavy usage over long time periods than had previously been thought (Falck et al. 2007).

Because of cocaine's stimulant effects on the noradrenergic system, heavy use carries significant risks of cardiovascular complications, including myocardial infarction and stroke, with high rates of these seen in the USA epidemic (Galanter et al. 1992, Pozner et al. 2005). Psychiatric effects are also common (Nnadi et al. 2005), including paranoid psychosis, which is well known among users; in heavy usage acute psychotic states can be severe and pose problems in containment of disturbed behaviour. Aggressiveness and violence frequently occur in such states and in craving for crack, when desperate measures may be adopted to obtain the drug. The crack dealing scene also seems to be a particularly violent one, notably associated with gun crime, and there are links between use by females and prostitution. Babies born to crack-using women may have specific abnormalities (Deltsidou 2001), and there is an increased risk of obstetric complications (Fajemirokun-Odudeyi & Lindow 2004).

As with other stimulant misusers, those who use cocaine will often also take various sedative drugs to 'come down', i.e. to terminate an episode and alleviate withdrawal effects. These have typically included cannabis, alcohol and benzodiazepines, but heroin is increasingly taken for this purpose by crack users, often to the point of becoming physically dependent on the opiate. A common stereotype used to be the crack user who is a dealer in heroin but never takes that drug himself, but at least in the UK these two forms of drug use are overlapping more, both within individuals and subculturally. Also use as a 'speedball' is common, i.e. simultaneous injection of crack and heroin in the same syringe (Rhodes et al. 2007).

The possible treatments for cocaine misuse and the evidence for their effectiveness have been the subject of many reviews (e.g. Withers et al. 1995, de Lima et al. 2002, O'Leary Hennessey et al. 2003, Preti 2007), and can be divided into pharmacological and non-pharmacological, or 'psychosocial'.

Pharmacological treatments

As cocaine abuse has risen in prominence and drug services have struggled to make an impact, it has often been suggested that the research priority must be to find a medication which is as effective in treating cocaine problems as methadone is in heroin dependence. This is portrayed as a quest which will eventually be fruitful, and yet in the absence of much serious consideration of the substitution model of treatment there is surely going to be no medication that fulfils the role of methadone or buprenorphine, with their routinely achievable benefits in heroin addicts due to the direct replacement in drug-taking. Rather, the investigations in cocaine abuse have mainly been into treatments which on biochemical grounds can be expected to alleviate withdrawal symptoms, or which might improve the condition in other more peripheral ways than drug substitution, such as stabilizing mood.

The classic description of cocaine withdrawal (Gawin & Kleber 1986) identified a syndrome in three stages: initially agitation, anorexia and acute craving; secondly excessive tiredness, depression and hyperphagia; and finally a normalization of most features but a return of craving when triggered by environmental cues. The euphoria produced by cocaine and the prominent withdrawal features of craving and depression are considered to be largely due to an increase, and then rebound depletion, in central dopamine transmission, and most early interest was in the dopaminergic drugs bromocriptine and amantadine, and the antidepressant desipramine, which acts substantially on dopamine transmission (Pollack et al. 1989). Controlled studies have mainly been of desipramine, with the findings of a meta-analysis indicating some benefit over placebo in promoting abstinence, but not in treatment retention, seemingly still valid (Levin & Lehman 1991, Preti 2007). To varying degrees, these three medications tend to be poorly tolerated, and studies have simply not been consistently positive (Soares et al. 2003). Carbamazepine has also been advocated (Halikas et al. 1997), on the basis that the withdrawal symptoms may represent minor convulsive phenomena, but again further controlled studies have not supported use of the drug.

An alternative approach with antidepressants is to use the specific serotonergic re-uptake inhibitors such as fluoxetine (Covi et al. 1995). Serotonin transmission is affected by cocaine in similar ways to that of dopamine, while other rationales for the use of these medications include quicker onset of action than the tricyclics, better acceptability, plus a possible effect in reducing drug craving which has been indicated in animal studies (Rothman & Baumann 2006) and in some amphetamine users (see page 90). Once again, however, the supporting evidence is quite weak (Grabowski et al. 1995, Moeller et al. 2007) and, with lithium and antipsychotic drugs also having been tried, there has recently been a flurry of interest in (perhaps surprisingly) disulfiram. In practice there are individuals who will usually manage to refrain from cocaine until they are disinhibited after drinking alcohol, and so disulfiram could have a role there in stopping the drinking in the first place, but actually a specific effect of the medication in modifying the reinforcing effects of cocaine has been claimed (Kampman 2008).

The approach of substitution treatment is not completely neglected in cocaine abuse, although the 'agonist therapies' which have mainly been tried are amphetamines rather than any cocaine product (Castells et al. 2007). Investigations have been small in scale, with possibly better reduction in cocaine use in individuals given a sustained-release amphetamine medication (Grabowski et al. 2001) than a short-acting form (Shearer et al. 2003). This kind of treatment is discussed further in the section on amphetamine prescribing in Chapter 2.

One of the most authoritative reviews of medications in cocaine abuse is by de Lima et al. (2002), and given the very large number of compounds which have been tried without good effect they advise that 'these time-consuming efforts [i.e. randomized trials] should be reserved for medications showing more relevant and promising evidence'. Certainly for clinicians faced with states of heavy compulsive crack use the prospects of medication making a significant impression can seem slight, sometimes with the exception of sedative antipsychotic drugs for agitation. In the presence of definite delusional symptoms full doses of a suitable antipsychotic may be required for a period, combined with efforts to prevent ongoing cocaine use. Benzodiazepines also have a limited role as symptomatic treatment in the acute stages of withdrawal (see page 54).

Finally, there are two experimental methods which have not yet been applied in ordinary or even specialized clinical practice. For a long time there has been interest in the prospect of vaccination, and while a variety of techniques have been used, the basic principle is that limited exposure to cocaine produces antibodies which then prevent full distribution of the drug into the brain if it is taken (Kantak 2003). The other approach, less researched, is to enhance drug excretion, to reduce the acute reinforcing effects of cocaine (Donovan et al. 2005).

Nonpharmacological treatments

Residential programmes and relapse prevention work for cocaine misusers often represent modified forms of treatment that is applicable across all substances (Weiss et al. 2005, Vaughan & McMahon 2006). Abstinence-based programmes such as twelve-step groups can contain a mix of users of various substances, and the place for this approach has not yet been usurped by any demonstrably more effective therapy, although there is currently much interest in some particular behavioural treatments.

One well-recognized feature of cocaine use is that withdrawal craving, and therefore risk of relapse, appears to be strongly 'cue-dependent' (van der Laar et al. 2004). Thus an individual may experience relatively few problems staying abstinent from cocaine in the early stages, until he or she encounters the particular situation in which they formerly used cocaine, when high arousal and strong cravings can occur. This makes an inpatient setting partly unrealistic for relapse prevention work, but in some units experimental situations have been set up where cues are simulated or drug paraphernalia presented, to work on the process of habituation (Conklin & Tiffany 2002).

Also in the realm of behaviour therapy but of a very different kind, many studies have investigated giving material incentives to cocaine users (and sometimes users of other drugs) in programmes as rewards for drug-free urines (Higgins et al. 2000, Rawson et al. 2006, Prendergast et al. 2006). Giving any kind of payments for abstaining from what was originally a 'deviant' behaviour attracts controversy, and certainly in the UK the media were very interested when this approach was approved in national guidelines, just as they are in situations such as school students being rewarded to attend correctly, or prisoners for doing constructive activities rather than watching television in their cells. In the drug programmes the incentives can be retail vouchers, money or 'clinic privileges', and it is unsurprising that better results have been shown with higher and prompter rewards (Petry 2006). Perhaps in the absence of the potent force of giving substitute medication in this form of drug misuse, the basic lure of money or equivalent is a suitably appealing alternative, and with the kinds of results demonstrated community services must take note and give material options serious consideration, even if applicability will vary across settings.

Other techniques showing positive results in studies include coping skills training, focusing on the analysis and practice of skills required in avoiding relapse (Rohsenow et al. 2004), cognitive therapy (Rawson et al. 2006), and various forms of individual and group drug counselling (Crits-Cristoph et al. 1999). There have been results of motivational enhancement therapy being more beneficial for patients with initial demonstrably low motivation than for those with higher levels (Rohsenow et al. 2004), while, as will now be discussed, broader service provision issues often need to be considered to engage more users even in the early steps towards treatment.

Practical management

Brief mention will be made here of a relatively large study carried out with my colleagues in Sheffield and Manchester after the first decade or so of extensive cocaine and crack use in the UK, which through survey methods and in-depth interviews, and then a follow-up of a cohort of patients in treatment, investigated the approaches which were being deployed in practice (Seivewright et al. 2000a). We had been commissioned to do this work by the Department of Health as it had become clear (as discussed above) that there was no consensus on any standard treatment, or even range of treatments, in cocaine abuse. The questionnaire survey was of drug misuse treatment services in England, and the in-depth interviews were with staff at services which had been successful in at least engaging relatively high proportions of cocaine misusers. Among a wide range of findings, some common themes emerged which were considered important in the management of cocaine misusers by workers across the range of disciplines. These are indicated in Table 4.2.

It was widely observed in this research that cocaine users were not inclined to attend services as they were delivered at the time, and there had been various initiatives to outreach to specific groups, including Afro-Caribbeans and women. Often cocaine users were given priority appointments, since attendance from a waiting list tended to be poor, one factor perhaps being the periodicity of usage. Where engagement was successful, counselling was mainly of a very practical nature, addressing immediate lifestyle problems and offering basic advice on harm reduction and methods of cutting down.

Table 4.2 Themes in treatment of cocaine misuse in England

Specific outreach
Prioritization
Practical counselling
Targeted use of pharmacological treatments
Admission in some severe cases
Acupuncture commonly used

Based on Seivewright et al. (2000a)

Pharmacological treatments were used by nearly half of the 149 services which offered any treatment, with a wide range of medications directed at various features of cocaine usage. Fluoxetine and desipramine were the most frequently prescribed antidepressants, with benzodiazepines used to aid sleep and reduce distress in withdrawal states. Sedative antipsychotics were used, apparently in states of severe agitation as well as more directly for psychotic complications.

Most staff interviewed had had experience of crack users presenting in states of heavy compulsive usage and great distress, such that admission of some kind was considered the only feasible option. Signs of physical or psychiatric illness would indicate hospital settings, but some rehabilitation centres accepted individuals whose main need appeared to be simply removal from availability of crack. The recourse to admission in acute situations highlighted the dearth of treatments definitely effective in reducing cocaine use, as in a different way did the generally widespread use of acupuncture and other alternative therapies. Of the complementary approaches, there is a degree of support for acupuncture from the literature, with possibly some specific sites relevant in stimulant misuse (Margolin 2003).

Case history

Darren is a 26-year-old man who was referred to our clinic as having problems with heroin and cocaine use. He was on probation following offences of robbery and assault, and a preliminary discussion with his probation officer indicated that crack cocaine had originally been Darren's drug of preference. His offences were related to his use of crack, at a time when he had been spending large amounts of money on the drug. Heroin use had gradually developed over the past year, and at two assessment appointments there were clinical signs of heroin use, and products of both drugs present in the urine.

The situation of daily dependent heroin use was sufficient to merit methadone treatment, but a (requested) detoxification attempt was not successful. His initial dosage was reinstated and the urine tests at his further appointments did not show heroin, but four consecutive tests showed cocaine, benzodiazepines and cannabis, in addition to his methadone. He was generally unenthusiastic about methadone, and after a pattern of missing an increasing number of collection days he dropped out of engagement with us.

Darren had also made contacts with a local street agency aimed at crack users, and he continued to see them frequently. Our next involvement was when we were asked to assess him in relation to funding for a stay at an out-of-town residential rehabilitation centre. It transpired that his situation had improved substantially, with a general reduction in drug use and temporary employment gained through a probation scheme. He claimed to no longer use opiates, but he would occasionally obtain tranquillizers and he sometimes drank heavily. He had made personal efforts, with support, to greatly reduce his use of crack, but he experienced strong cravings, and his mood was frequently low. There were clinical grounds for prescribing an antidepressant, and he was given fluoxetine 20 mg per day, and reviewed at a short series of appointments. He reports some reduction in craving and improvement in mood, and urine sampling accords with his self-reported reductions in drug use. He was approved for residential treatment, but at present he does not wish to take this up because of his job, and because he feels he can manage without it.

Cocaine misuse by opioid substitution patients

One form of cocaine misuse which is encountered frequently in services is the additional use of the drug by patients on methadone or buprenorphine. In areas of high cocaine availability it should simply never be a surprise to practitioners to see this combination, with the most basic explanation being that treatment with an opioid substitute has much less effect on non-opiate use than opiate use. Many studies have shown high rates of cocaine use in drug users on entry to programmes (e.g. Grella et al. 1997, Gossop et al. 2002a, b), but several have also found that as patients at least manage to abstain reasonably satisfactorily from heroin when on their opioid, a switch can occur to cocaine as the illicit drug of choice, with usage increasing or even starting newly after programme entry (Chaisson et al. 1989, Gossop et al. 2002, Williamson et al. 2006). Part of the effectiveness of methadone or buprenorphine is to remove the financial and social complications of users spending money and commiting crime for heroin, but the behavioural patterns of using money for drugs and seeking intoxication often do not go away in any short timescale. In various ways cocaine abuse during opioid substitution treatments can be a fairly direct result of the intervention, and so doctors who are willing to prescribe extensively to addicts must also have knowledge of the more complicated field of managing cocaine abuse.

Although small scale, we had a clear illustration of the above situation when a student on attachment in our service systematically investigated the use of cocaine by methadone and buprenorphine patients, at one point enquiring in non-clinic interviews whether patients' use of heroin and cocaine respectively had been less, about the same, or increased since starting on treatment (Seivewright et al. 2006). The contrast is shown in Figure 4.1, with all except one of the individuals who had been using heroin reporting a decrease since starting their opioid, but in those who had used cocaine more people reporting similar or actually increased usage since treatment than reduced use.

For policy reasons which will be well known to many readers and which have to an extent been rehearsed in this book, fewer and fewer programmes will now discharge patients for persistent drug use on top of their prescribed medication, instead prioritizing continued engagement and harm reduction. It is therefore inevitable that the situation of additional cocaine use will need to be managed, and broadly speaking it is the specific treatments which have been tried in primary cocaine abuse and which have been reviewed above which need to be attempted. Once again contingency management, with various kinds of rewards for cocaine-free urines, has been among the most successful approaches (Dallery et al. 2001, Rowan-Szal et al. 2005), with more equivocal results for other psychological treatments. Additional antidepressants including fluoxetine or desipramine seem often unhelpful, while the prescribing of dexamphetamine has possibly more effect (Grabowski et al. 2004).

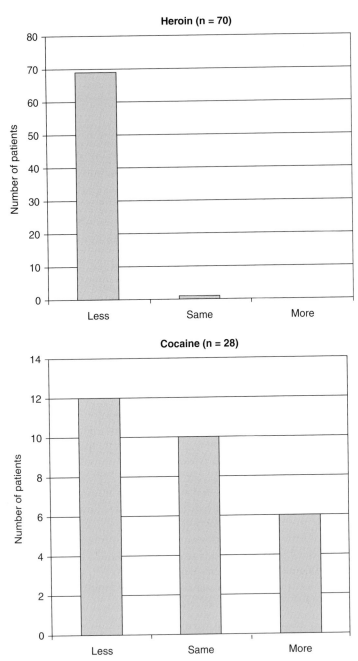

Figure 4.1 Reported use of drugs by patients after starting on opioid substitution treatment (*n* = 72).

The important difference in the cocaine-abusing opioid patient scenario is that there is also the dose of methadone, buprenorphine or alternative to consider, and there seems little doubt in practice and from study results that at least some individuals will refrain from other drug use better if their opioid is increased (Faggiano et al. 2004).

As for any difference between the rates of cocaine abuse in individuals on methadone and buprenorphine, there is a theoretical consideration that perhaps less cocaine use can be expected on the latter because of a reduced mutually reinforcing ('speedball') effect with only partial opioid agonist activity, and some empirical support for this (Foltin & Fischman 1996, Giacomuzzi et al. 2003). However, Schottenfeld et al. (2005) found superiority of methadone over buprenorphine in treatment retention and periods of abstinence in their cocaine-abusing opioid patients.

As indicated earlier, a proportion of crack users who use heroin to 'come down' from their drug become dependent enough on the opiate for methadone or buprenorphine to be considered. In such cases of true dual dependency, opioid substitution may offer the best chance of a stabilizing effect on drug use and lifestyle, but the same rules of treatment need to be applied as to any other opioid patient. In practice, progress in those who were initially crack users tends to be problematic, with difficulties in abstaining from the favoured drug, and often poor acceptance of methadone's effects. Further expertise needs to be gained with this group, and the situation must be avoided whereby methadone is simply offering an alternative sedative to those previously used, with little impact on stimulant use.

Overall, therefore, as with cocaine abuse in general there is much theory to draw on when managing cocaine-misusing methadone or buprenorphine patients, but often difficulties in the clinical situation. Some feel that the move towards 'harm reduction' opioid prescribing has made it virtually impossible to counter a switch to stimulant usage which a patient may claim to be 'recreational'. However, it seems advisable to adopt a reasonably assertive approach within clinic appointments, and in our own practice the urine drug screening results (with there being testing at every appointment) are used as a focus for discussion, even if only briefly. Cocaine only remains detectable for a very short period – often one to two days – after usage, and so it is right to tactfully counter a claim by an individual that their use of the drug is 'occasional' when it is present in every sample. We have completely lost count of the occasions when we have been told that the sample results are unlucky, because the patient receives their welfare money on, say, a Thursday and our appointments are on Fridays! However, it is entirely legitimate to make observations about the implications of using the family welfare money on additional drug use, along with advice on the risks of cocaine, and in this way it is easy to see how 'feedback of results' is considered by some to be an actual behavioural therapy. Sometimes such feedback is used as a control intervention in comparative studies with a more specific behavioural treatment, for instance contingency management (Schottenfeld et al. 2005). A basic but important use of contingency management principles is also very common and seemingly effective in practice, i.e. progressing to more 'take-home' opioid dosing and less frequent clinic attendance as abstinence from cocaine improves.

Topic in brief – 9. Cocaine use by opioid substitution patients

- Methadone and buprenorphine reduce opiate use far more than non-opiate use
- A switch to cocaine or other substances should be anticipated on behavioural grounds
- Claims that use is occasional or unproblematic need to be tested
- Behaviour therapies range from feedback of results to systematic contingency management
- As with primary cocaine use, specific medications relatively ineffective

Amphetamine

There is an extraordinary lack of literature on the treatment of amphetamine problems, with this subject almost universally regarded by observers in the UK as an unjustly neglected area. Use of the drug is hugely widespread but, as with cocaine, voluntary presentation to services other than needle exchange is at a low rate. Amphetamine misuse does not have the same media profile as that of cocaine, and yet the reasons for which services were exhorted to engage large numbers of drug users at the time of the HIV crisis would appear to be particularly pertinent to this group. The frustrations that were well voiced by Klee (1992), who referred to amphetamine use as 'a case study in neglect', in which the 'myopic focus on the casualties of heroin' has led to amphetamine problems 'not being taken seriously', still apply. That author presented comparative data showing higher rates of HIV-risk-taking behaviours in injecting amphetamine users than heroin users, and pointed to the many studies indicating high levels of sexual activity.

With studies of treatment few and far between, the general forms of management have been discussed from a UK perspective by Myles (1997) and by ourselves (Seivewright et al. 2005). The use of harm-reduction measures, general and specialized counseling (Baker et al. 2005) and pharmacological treatments for withdrawal features or psychiatric complications may be seen as basically similar to the application of the same approaches in cocaine misuse, while in drug services there has been interest in two particular treatment aspects. In a series of cases Polson et al. (1993) found that fluoxetine, in ordinary dosage of 20 mg per day, helped some amphetamine users cut down or stop their drug. The medication was given for two weeks in the first instance, with counselling therapies where indicated. This evidence is basically no stronger than that for the same medication in cocaine misuse, but in the absence of definite other options the strategy has been quite widely taken up by services which see significant numbers of amphetamine users. Given the other evidence for serotonergic compounds reducing drug-seeking (Burmeister et al. 2003) and appetitive and compulsive behaviours, it certainly seems reasonable to select a medication of this type if significant persistent depression in a stimulant user suggests an antidepressant. The second treatment approach which is being used is more controversial, namely limited substitute prescribing with dexamphetamine sulphate (McBride et al. 1997, Shearer et al. 2001, Merrill et al. 2005). Many specialists in the UK consider that, although a substitution approach is inherently much less satisfactory in amphetamine users than opiate users for various clinical reasons, it is not necessary to rule it out completely, and they will prescribe in some cases of severe dependence. This issue is discussed in detail in Chapter 2.

The treatment options for amphetamine users in our own community services which have developed pragmatically over the years are summarized in Table 4.3.

Most amphetamine users purely receive behaviourally based drug counselling, covering the aspects described in the section on general counselling in Chapter 5. This includes all individuals whose use of amphetamine, in either the powder form or increasingly the rather purer 'base', is short-term and/or occasional (e.g. weekends), and those in whom there is no convincing indication for pharmacological treatments. Beyond simply weekend use, other users take the drug for a run of a few days, until some over-agitation and paranoid experiences signal the time to stop and catch up on eating and sleeping. In counselling, such users are specifically encouraged to increase their drug-free days, and advised on behavioural tactics which can help in doing this. Good background evidence for effectiveness of cognitive-behavioural therapy in such usage is provided by Feeney et al. (2006), with the

Table 4.3 A scheme for community treatment of amphetamine misuse

Treatment	Indications
Counselling alone	Short-term use (< 6 months)
	Occasional use
	Not injecting
Counselling plus limited course of symptomatic medication: fluoxetine, diazepam, hypnotics	Inability to otherwise tolerate withdrawal effects
Counselling plus dexamphetamine sulphate prescribing	Heavy daily injected use
	Severe direct health or social problems
	Other approaches failed but motivation to avoid illicit amphetamine is high

counselling focusing on refusal self-efficacy, improved coping, improved problem-solving and planning for relapse prevention.

The next category of treatment comprises drug counselling plus symptomatic medication, and is for those who want to stop their usage but have found themselves unable to do so through not being able to tolerate the withdrawal effects. Many such individuals use amphetamine on most days, and they may have progressed to injecting. Amphetamine withdrawal features are usually considered to primarily include depression, hypersomnia and hyperphagia, with debate as to whether these constitute a syndrome as such, or simply represent the rebound effects of the drug's actions. Many relatively heavy users who attempt to stop, however, experience a more complex combination of symptoms: irritability and aggressiveness are frequent and may partly represent a personality-determined response to discomfort, while there are often various aches and pains, anxiety and craving, with insomnia occurring after two or three days if the withdrawal attempt lasts that far. In a well-motivated individual who has experienced such difficulties, we prescribe diazepam and/or a non-benzodiazepine hypnotic such as zopiclone in ordinary dosage in a one- to two-week course, plus fluoxetine 20 mg per day. Such prescribing is satisfactory only if it is part of a concentrated and supported effort to abstain, but with good community supervision the alleviation of symptoms, notably insomnia, can enable successful withdrawal. Benzodiazepines must be clearly time-limited to avoid dependence, but fluoxetine may be continued for the length of a normal antidepressant course if there are sufficient grounds.

Prescribing of dexamphetamine sulphate is considered only in the most severe cases of dependence, such as individuals using of the order of 7 grams per day, injecting several times a day, often with a history dating back many years. There must not only be demonstrable severe health or social problems produced by such use, but the individual must be motivated to greatly modify or preferably stop their use of street amphetamine if taken on for prescribing. Like other services, although we would rather prescribe on the basis of complete abstinence, we have had cases where intravenous use is so heavy that prescribing has been effectively on harm-reduction grounds (just as is routinely accepted in the management of opioid dependence). General criteria, monitoring and prescribing methods are as described in Chapter 2, where there is a case history from our service. At the levels of street amphetamine usage for which we prescribe, a starting dose of 60 mg per day of dexamphetamine sulphate mixture is usually required; this is considered a maximum, so that if prescribing were done exceptionally for a person using only 2–3 grams per day, the daily dexamphetamine dose could be 40 mg. Dispensing is daily or two to three times per week, with gradual reductions in dosage and/or in the number of days on which medication is taken in a week. We prescribe for a maximum of six months, and so the aim is for full reduction during this time. When prescribing is purely on a harm-reduction basis, the same maximum period is applied, in which case repeat courses may be necessary after a period, with the user strongly encouraged to move towards reduction and abstinence.

Many drug services in the UK (Klee et al. 2001) and other countries (e.g. Lintzeris et al. 1996) have provided treatment for amphetamine users along similar lines to the above overall scheme. Systematic and assertive drug counselling should be the basis of treatment, and where efforts are directed at engaging more amphetamine users, it should primarily be with that aim and to provide the direct harm-reduction measures such as injecting equipment provision. The prescribing element attracts the controversy, and is sometimes over-emphasized in terms of promoting engagement, but in the present state of evidence this can only be considered suitable for a very small proportion of cases.

Case history

Robert is 28 years old and had used drugs since teenage years. For many years his preference was amphetamines, progressing to daily injected use. He then moved on to using heroin, presenting to our service about a year later. He completed a community detoxification from heroin but, perhaps predictably, relapsed into amphetamine use. He was re-referred by the probation service after committing several offences.

At this time Robert was injecting amphetamine several times a day, and was living in a house with other amphetamine users. He had clearly become paranoid, believing the television was referring to him, and generally avoiding people.

The drug worker who knew Robert from before took on his case, and saw him for a series of appointments. Counselling emphasized that the time was right to give up amphetamine, as his family had become very concerned and were willing to support him. He was helped to become aware that amphetamine was causing his mental symptoms, and he was systematically encouraged to have drug-free days, on an increasing basis.

In just three weeks Robert stopped using amphetamine, with no medication necessary. In view of the progress he had made, he was given support and assistance in finding accommodation of his own. His paranoid symptoms resolved, to the extent that he volunteered information to the police to clear up some previous charges. Three months on, there has been no relapse and no new offending behaviour.

Methylenedioxymethamphetamine (MDMA, 'ecstasy')

This is the drug which had such a strong influence in the nightclub culture in many countries through the 1990s. With semihallucinogenic effects in addition to the stimulant amphetamine actions, it has been associated with a revival of 'psychedelia', to some extent recalling the use of LSD in the 1960s. The distinctive setting for using ecstasy is at a 'rave', typically all-night, with characteristic repetitive and energetic music and dancing. Taking ecstasy or an alternative stimulant or hallucinogen became almost an integral part of the rave experience (Boys et al. 1997), and in youth culture in the UK at the time this represented the most significant new wave of drug-taking since the advent of smokable heroin. Amphetamine and LSD are commonly used by the same individuals and groups, while there are many slight chemical variants of ecstasy, such as methylenedioxyethylamphetamine (MDEA, 'eve'), and unrelated chemicals are sometimes marketed as ecstasy, such as ketamine. In the new century it appears that the prevalence of ecstasy use may be declining, with a rise instead in the use of cocaine by the young.

In general the modern usage of ecstasy has been characterized by higher doses and/or more frequent consumption than were typical in a previous era of recreational use of the drug in the USA (Peroutka et al. 1988, Baylen & Rosenberg 2006). That earlier usage owed something to a legal (at the time) use in psychotherapy, and appears to have been generally fairly restrained, although widespread, particularly among college students. Alongside the desired effects, a range of minor adverse effects were recognized, some of which resembled those of amphetamine, including anorexia, and irritability and depression on stopping the drug. Some were slightly more characteristic, such as jaw tension and teeth grinding, but the major problems only emerged as usage became generally heavier and associated with the nightclub scene.

The most severe adverse effects are unexpected deaths and a range of psychiatric complications, and in both cases there is a limited understanding of aetiology (Cole & Sumnall 2003, Thomasius et al. 2003). The sudden deaths have often followed the development of hyperthermia, with features such as disseminated intravascular coagulation, rhabdomyolysis and acute renal failure (Henry et al. 1992). Dosage in these individual instances seems of limited relevance, with some deaths having occurred after just one tablet, and the hot environmental conditions in nightclubs have been implicated. Spontaneous intracerebral haemorrhage has also been reported, while of the nonfatal complications a toxic hepatitis may relate partly to contaminants.

The connection between ecstasy use and a range of alleged psychiatric adverse effects is difficult to ascertain. Beyond the minor depressive reactions which are common after stimulants (and can cause absenteeism after weekend ecstasy use), other conditions which appear possible complications include anxiety and panic disorders, more severe depression, psychoses and flashback experiences. The evidence from case reports has been gathered together by Soar et al. (2001), while the links appear quite strong in some systematic research, reviewed by Thomasius et al. (2005). Pre-existing vulnerability to psychiatric or physical conditions is often suggested as an explanation of why only a small proportion of users suffer serious ill-effects, but there are also striking reports of severe symptoms persisting in previously healthy individuals long after use of the drug (e.g. Soar et al. 2004). In general, it may be relevant that ecstasy and related compounds are known to be neurotoxic to serotonergic neurons in various animals including primates (Colado et al. 2004), although the significance of associated abnormalities which have been demonstrated in humans is as yet uncertain (Parrot 2004, Gouzoulis-Mayfrank & Daumann 2006). In a post-mortem study a range of neuropathological changes in the brain have been demonstrated, along with various organ toxicity effects, in individuals who had taken ecstasy or MDEA (Milroy et al. 1996).

With ecstasy users rarely presenting to treatment services other than after the development of complications, the management of this form of drug misuse has mainly been in the harm-reduction arena. Because dehydration appears important in the potentially fatal physical effects, there has been much advice for users at raves regarding measures such as taking rest periods and maintaining an adequate fluid intake, with organizers being required to make suitable conditions available. Unfortunately the perils of giving advice of this kind have been brought home by the knowledge that some deaths have involved dilutional effects of overhydration, which has left the harm-reduction situation in some confusion. It seems that the recommendations regarding amounts of fluid to drink have been broadly correct, but that some individuals may develop a kind of compulsive drinking, which it is known can occur with amphetamine misuse.

Treatment of psychiatric complications should generally be along standard lines for the respective conditions. Some syndromes appear to be brief and self-limiting once ecstasy use stops, but a more chronic course may also be seen, with cases in the literature of psychoses which prove resistant to treatment (Vecellio et al. 2003). Whichever psychiatric syndrome occurs, there is possibly a theoretical indication for specific serotonergic re-uptake inhibitors such as fluoxetine, sertraline or citalopram, given the effect of ecstasy in reducing serotonin transmission. This would purely be a pragmatic approach which has not yet been properly tested, and it may be that the transmission abnormalities are not amenable to this kind of enhancement.

Case history

Paul was referred by his general practitioner to our clinic, at 29 years old with no previous contact. He was a successful businessman, and lived in a desirable residential area with his parents. He drank alcohol in moderation, and until recently his only drug use was smoking cannabis on a handful of occasions.

Two months before presenting to his doctor, Paul had used ecstasy twice at a nightclub, about a week apart. He reported that he had 'not felt right since', experiencing anxiety and some more severe panic attacks. He had been unable to concentrate at work, and generally felt he was functioning poorly. He had palpitations on any significant exertion, and had little energy. Over the period he had felt increasingly depressed, wondering what was happening to him and sometimes breaking down in tears. His appetite was poor and he had lost some weight.

It was considered that his symptoms could be directly due to ecstasy, but also that some secondary anxiety and depression were likely. For short-term symptom relief he was pre-scribed diazepam 2mg tablets up to four per day for one week. He was also given citalopram 20mg per day, and the need to avoid ecstasy or any illicit drugs was reinforced.

Paul's various symptoms improved slowly over the course of about three months. Sometimes his anxiety would become more prominent, and very limited further supplies of diazepam were given. The improvement in mood was also not dramatic, with the effect of medication uncertain. He is now on no medication, and feels virtually back to his 'old self'. He is sure that he will not use ecstasy or any other drugs again and, with the increased risk through anxiety, he has been advised not to increase his alcohol intake.

Methamphetamine ('crystal meth', 'ice')

Although the terminology can be confusing, especially in laboratory analyses for 'meth-amphetamines' which can include ecstasy, the drug known actually as methamphetamine with the above alternative names is a separate preparation currently causing much concern. High rates of use have been found in the USA, various parts of Asia and also Eastern European countries, while in the UK for a few years there has been relatively confined use in nightclubs in metropolitan centres. The potency of the drug appears to result in quite frequent amphetamine-type complications including psychosis (McKetin et al. 2006), with treatment efforts being in relatively early stages (e.g. Vocci and Appel 2007). At the time of writing there are no specific treatments to be recommended, while international efforts at control continue (Ghodse 2007).

Khat

This is a plant product with amphetamine-like effects, leaves and twigs of which are chewed mainly by inhabitants or expatriates of Somalia and neighbouring East African and Arab countries. Undoubtedly the same stimulation, anorexia and weight loss and psychiatric effects can occur as from amphetamine use, but there is little guidance on any effective treatment. A fascinating review has been provided from the Oral Microbiology department at Bergen University (Al-Hebshi & Skaug 2005), covering not only the scientific aspects but also details of social context of usage.

Benzodiazepines

Benzodiazepine problems are often thought of as relating to individuals with minor psychiatric disorders, literally millions of whom have become dependent after being prescribed the drugs in ordinary dosage (Lader 1993). Clear-cut demonstrations of physical dependence in controlled studies occurred some two decades after the drugs had been introduced (Tyrer et al. 1981, Petursson & Lader 1981), and there has been much criticism in retrospect of the over-prescribing of benzodiazepines in situations such as adjustment reactions or bereavement, and now also of the lack of treatment services for this group. Individuals dependent on prescribed benzodiazepines are reluctant to attend drug misuse services with their emphasis on illicit drug use, injecting and HIV, although some such services have separate support groups. Much of the management of benzodiazepine withdrawal takes place in primary care practice, and the usual approach, comprising preparation, transfer to a long-acting benzodiazepine, graded withdrawal, and sometimes additional counselling or pharmacological treatments, has been described in practical reviews (Lader & Morton 1991, Mant & Walsh 1997, Oude Voshaar et al. 2006).

While some individuals who are prescribed benzodiazepines in ordinary circumstances increase their dosage to develop a form of definite misuse (van Valkenburg & Akiskal 1999), the problems of benzodiazepine misuse by polydrug users are often very different in nature (Seivewright 1998, Darke et al. 2002). Studies have mainly been of prevalence and patterns of misuse, usually carried out in drug treatment settings such as methadone clinics, but with little examination of management of benzodiazepine misuse itself. Diazepam has been shown to enhance the subjective effects of opiates (Preston et al. 1984), and in one clinical survey most methadone maintenance patients who used diazepam reportedly took it within an hour of taking their methadone for that reason (Stitzer et al. 1981), although in practice usage later in the day to prolong a lowish dose of methadone also seems common. Benzodiazepines are frequently taken by stimulant misusers (Darke et al. 1994a), partly to alleviate stimulant withdrawal effects, and by drug misusers with a preference for the similar effects of alcohol, or they may be a primary drug of misuse, relatively rarely in terms of presentation to treatment services. Prevalence rates of benzodiazepine use in polydrug users are high (Iguchi et al. 1993, Ross et al. 1997, Nielsen et al. 2007), up to 94% for lifetime use, with rates in studies largely determined by timescale and type of population investigated.

In the UK there has been particular concern over injected benzodiazepine misuse, usually of temazepam, which in the 1980s was formulated as a capsule with liquid content which could be extracted. This form of drug misuse produced severe psychological consequences such as amnesia and disturbed or aggressive behaviour (Ruben & Morrison 1992), and direct complications of injection leading to amputations were frequent. The formulation was changed to a thicker gel content, but allegations followed that this had made matters worse, in that if drug misusers persisted in injecting temazepam the local effects seemed more severe. This was not clearly proved, but the drug has now been assigned to a higher level of control than the other benzodiazepines in the UK, and its prescription to drug misusers is generally discouraged. Because of the continued association of temazepam, even in the now usual tablet form, with high dose and injected misuse, in our own clinics we will not include this particular benzodiazepine in any of our prescribing regimes (see Chapter 2). The injection of benzodiazepines by illicit drug users in Australia in a period after the UK's height of usage has also been examined (Darke et al. 2002).

The temazepam phenomenon is an example of a very harmful form of benzodiazepine use by illicit drug users, but we may presume that overall there is a wide spectrum of harm of usage with, at the lower end, occasional moderate oral use which may be unproblematic. Nevertheless, in a series of formative investigations Darke and colleagues (Darke et al. 1992b, 1993, 1994a) found benzodiazepine use in polydrug users to be associated with a range of adverse physical, psychological and social features, suggesting both problems of a direct nature and also perhaps that benzodiazepine use may generally be an indicator of more severe drug misuse. One of the features consistently detected was increased HIV-risk behaviours, which fits with a study in which temazepam use was found to be strongly associated with a range of high-risk injecting and sexual practices (Klee et al. 1990). The possible explanations there appeared to be that either individuals who indulged in risky behaviours were selectively attracted to temazepam, or that some result of taking temazepam, such as the amnesia or confusion, produced the high-risk practices. Although the implications of a study of injecting temazepam users cannot be extrapolated to other situations, there is ongoing concern about the sheer extent to which drug misusers obtain benzodiazepines from general practitioners, with such consultations and prescribing being vastly more common than among the general population (Darke et al. 2003).

The most direct form of treatment of benzodiazepine misuse, deriving from the literature on ordinary-dose dependence, is detoxification where indicated, and this has been discussed in Chapter 2. Also highlighted there are the great difficulties in practice in agreeing suitable regimes with habitual users, who are often used to taking high doses and indeed may well have been obtaining tranquillizers from a range of sources (Nielsen et al. 2007). Doctors are no doubt sometimes fearful that severe withdrawal symptoms such as fits could possibly occur if prescribing is not done, but much pressure is also applied by drug misusers, and readily giving out tranquillizers probably causes more problems overall than it solves. Again as previously indicated it should always be borne in mind that the prevalence of actual physical dependence on benzodiazepines in illicit users is relatively low (Williams et al. 1996, Ross & Darke 2000), and that in observed situations control can readily be gained by low-dose and short-term prescribing.

There have unfortunately been very few systematic examinations of treatment of benzodiazepine misuse or dependence in the illicit drug population, and knowledge on the subject has been rather static over the last decade or so. When special programmes are tried the difficulties which seem inherent in this area are still apparent, such as in the randomized controlled study of reducing benzodiazepine dosing and cognitive behavioural therapy versus standard treatment by Vorma et al. (2002). The subjects were outpatients in clinics for alcohol and drug abusers, and strong benefit of the therapy was found, but with cessation of benzodiazepine use only occurring in small numbers. It might be observed that there is not enough consensus on managing this form of drug misuse for 'standard treatment' to be definable, and it is of interest that the paper states this was a

gradual benzodiazepine taper scheduled and managed by a physician and discussions with a nurse or therapist. The researchers did not define the rate of the taper or themes of the discussions beforehand. Diaries of benzodiazepine doses were used as a basis for dose reductions [and] the individual nurses and therapists applied their customary approaches, which were mainly supportive, and in some cases brief psychotherapy with strength perspective and using focused problem-solving techniques.

This probably reflects a common range of methods in practice, although from our own experience I would add that it seems better not to allow too much (or any) prior discussion of forthcoming reductions in dosage, as many reasons tend to be given to avoid these! Again as examined in Chapter 2 there is virtually no support for benzodiazepine 'maintenance' as there is for that with methadone and buprenorphine, and almost certainly benzodiazepines are far more often diverted to others than the opioid substitutes whose consumption can be supervised, with in the worst cases the tablets representing little more than currency.

Because benzodiazepines can be prescribed and because there is a demonstrable withdrawal syndrome there is inevitably a focus on this method of managing dependence, but there is also the parallel aim of rendering an individual drug-free, just as there would be if their additional drug of preference was cocaine rather than tranquillizers. A long time ago the principles of contingency management were applied to methadone patients who additionally used benzodiazepines (Stitzer et al. 1982), and 'clinic privileges' can undoubtedly be linked to clean urines in this as in other forms of polydrug use.

Cyclizine

The previous edition of this book contained a detailed description of abuse of the antiemetic tablet preparation cyclizine by illicit drug users, nearly always crushed and injected along with methadone tablets or ampoules. Cyclizine is a constituent of Diconal along with the opioid dipipanone, and it seems that cyclizine has an opioid-enhancing effect which partly accounts for the particularly euphoriant property of Diconal. This could therefore be reproduced by combining cyclizine with the synthetic opioid methadone, and the intention to do this led to a wave of patients in the UK attempting to have their methadone prescribed in the ampoule or tablet form.

The main study of this phenomenon was by Ruben et al. (1989), and there has been little further information, with cyclizine abuse seemingly declining as the national guidelines on methadone prescribing have increasingly opposed the use of non-mixture forms. Those of us working in areas of high prevalence of cyclizine abuse saw many complications, ranging from extreme confusion, neuromuscular twitching and a bizarre startled appearance in habitual users, to particularly severe problems from injecting and indeed post-mortem findings where the lungs were heavy from the residue of injected tablets. The clinical lesson is definitely that cyclizine should not be prescribed to drug misusers or individuals with a history which is even suggestive of that, whatever the claimed indication.

Hallucinogens

Hallucinogenic mushrooms, containing psilocybin, and lysergic acid diethylamide (LSD) are extremely common recreational drugs. Like ecstasy and related drugs, LSD has a strong affinity at various types of serotonin receptors in the brain, and it is conceivable that serotonergic compounds could have some role in modifying the effects of LSD (O'Brien 1996). In practice, the times these forms of drug misuse are encountered by clinical services are when there are additional mental effects, such as acute confusional states, anxiety reactions or psychotic features. In relation to such aspects, it should be noted that many papers on LSD relate to usage in the early times of modern recreational drug use, i.e. the 1960s and 70s, when much stronger preparations of the drug were taken than is the case now. Our own department has undertaken a more recent review of clinical aspects of mushroom use (Seivewright & Lagundoye 2007).

Hallucinogens may worsen pre-existing mental disorders, and the implications in relation to psychoses are discussed in Chapter 7. There is particular debate about the status of 'flashback experiences', unwanted recurrences of drug effects which appear to occur for some time after use of LSD, and also cannabis. A thorough review of the psychiatric adverse effects of LSD (Abraham & Aldridge 1993) found strong supportive evidence for panic reactions, prolonged schizoaffective psychoses and flashbacks, or more constant 'post-hallucinogen perceptual disorder', the latter continuing for as long as five years. Treatments which have occasionally been recommended for perceptual disturbances include halo-peridol, simple reassurance and short-term benzodiazepines.

Steroids

The patterns of anabolic–androgenic steroid use by sportspeople and body-builders, and their physical and psychological side-effects and dependence potential, have been very well reviewed by Brower (2002). Much of the use is by injection, and so many of this population attend needle exchanges, with the advice on reducing infection risks relevant. To increase energy, burn fat and to go through the 'pain barrier' some will use amphetamines and opiates, either street preparations or illicit pharmaceutical supplies. In the UK the opioid nalbuphine (Nubain) has been abused in this way and, in cases where dependence becomes established, detoxification treatments can be necessary.

While much of the interest with steroids is in their detection and control within sport, as clinicians we will particularly see those who have become opiate-dependent through nalbuphine. In many ways the management of these individuals resembles treatment of those dependent on the so-called minor opioids, with typically resistance to the idea of attending methadone clinics or having daily supervised consumption in a pharmacy. Often buprenorphine seems a good option, and in practice there may well be more 'take-home' dosing allowed as there are usually fewer complications of additional illicit drug use. It may be that in this population who have not had long-term dependence on opiates, detoxification courses will be sufficient more often than in the primary heroin users, but there is not systematic data on this and sometimes ongoing prescribing can be indicated.

Volatile substances

This is another of the forms of drug misuse which has been studied extensively from a phenomenological point of view, but for which there are few significant treatment avenues. It is known to be hazardous and potentially fatal through several mechanisms, including anoxia and heart arrhythmias (Ridenour 2005), with many deaths occurring after inhalation of cigarette lighter refills, aerosols and glues. The trends in casualties have shown changes in relation to substances as successive controls have been introduced, rather than overall reductions, indicating the difficulty in addressing the underlying tendency towards adolescent substance misuse. The majority of deaths are consistently in males under 20 years old, with substantial proportions occurring in first-time or near first-time users, sometimes through 'sudden sniffing death' or accidents when intoxicated. More committed solvent misuse is also problematic in other ways, being strongly linked with various forms of depression (Evren et al. 2006) and with conduct disorders and other behavioural and social problems (Lubman et al. 2006).

The general management approach to this form of drug misuse is preventive. A small subgroup of users, however, become truly dependent, for instance inhaling glue every 15 minutes of each day for long periods so that the problem dominates their life, and treatment attempts must be made with these individuals. Some rehabilitation centres will take such cases, and a 'detoxification' may be feasible, usually as an inpatient, with sedative medications used to alleviate distress. Practical advice for less severe cases is inevitably along harm-reduction lines, addressing for instance circumstances of usage, while the broader methods of tackling the problem have been reviewed by the UK's Advisory Council on the Misuse of Drugs (1995), and by Lubman et al. (2006) in Australia. Specific psychological or psychiatric treatment may be indicated in some cases, including antidepressants.

Cannabis

There is always plenty of controversy on the subject of cannabis, given the sheer extent of usage and the continuing view that, even with evidence of some of the consequent health problems becoming stronger in recent times, the drug is still one of the less harmful among those currently illegal in the UK and elsewhere. Those favouring decriminalization point out for comparison the hazards of the legally sanctioned alcohol and tobacco, and claim that the alleged progression on to other drugs would actually be less likely if cannabis did not have to be bought from dealers. They feel it a waste of police time to be occupied with cannabis offences, which make up a huge proportion of total drug offences, and indeed in the UK possession of the drug is usually dealt with by caution only. The opposing view is that hazards of present substances are not a reason to introduce a further one, and that the illegal status presumably acts as some deterrent to more widespread use of a drug which does have very significant adverse effects.

In UK drug services virtually all those dependent on opiates and other 'harder' drugs have used cannabis, but of course that does not answer the question that a lot of people are interested in, the proportion of cannabis users who make the progression. What is very common in presenting patients is a 'hierarchy' of the type most clearly demonstrated by Kandel and Davies (1992), with alcohol and tobacco typically preceding cannabis, which in turn preceded use of hallucinogens and 'pills' and, in a minority, later use of heroin and cocaine. That work was in America but a similar pattern is seen in many countries, and the related finding that early age of first taking cannabis, and heavy use, were associated with the subsequent use of heroin and cocaine also seems very applicable. Patterns of these kinds have indeed been further demonstrated (e.g. Wagner & Anthony 2002), with emphasis also on the importance of intial exposure to the various drugs, which varies not just between different countries but between males and females.

The psychological and physical adverse effects of cannabis have been the subject of many studies, with psychological ones in particular much debated (Hall & Solowij 2006). The suspicion of an 'amotivational syndrome' has not exactly gone away, but it seems such an entity cannot be distinguished from common personality characteristics among cannabis users, and the effects of chronic intoxication (Hall & Solowij 1997, 2006). Similarly, heavy cannabis use itself, rather than additional adverse effects, is likely to account for findings of cognitive impairment in long-term users. The evidence for increased risk of psychosis has recently become much more convincing, and indeed lay behind calls for a reclassification of cannabis to a higher level of control in the UK, just shortly after its status had been lowered by the government. Many experts feel that it is not quite possible yet to conclude that cannabis can directly produce psychosis in individuals with no recognized vulnerability features at all (Verdoux 2004, and see Chapter 7). However, between 2002 and 2005 a total of ten longitudinal studies were published which have been very influential, particularly the re-examination of data from over 50 000 Swedish males in the army who had originally been studied for the same reason by Andreasson et al. (1987) (Zammit et al. 2002). In a 27-year follow-up the authors concluded that cannabis use was associated with a substantially increased risk of developing schizophrenia, and that this risk was related to extent of usage. The association could not be explained by use of other psychoactive substances or medications or personality traits, and similar findings from other recent studies have been reviewed by Ben Amar and Potvin (2007). Although some of the cannabis use in those investigations was distant, there seems little doubt currently that the increasing strength of many intensively grown cannabis products is relevant in psychiatric disturbances, with the actual amount of tetrahydrocannabinol in plants having been described as 'the forgotten variable' (Smith 2005). An excellent critical analysis of the evidence on cannabis and psychosis has been provided by Fergusson et al. (2006).

Mood disturbances such as depression and anxiety may again, in different cases or in part, reflect underlying predisposition or the effects of usage (Moore et al. 2007), with Troisi et al. (1998) demonstrating a strong relationship between prevalence of psychiatric disorders and extent of actual cannabis dependence. More direct usage effects are psychomotor impairments, of the kinds which impair driving ability for a period. Respiratory diseases relate to smoking as the method of administration, while there is possibly increased risk of upper digestive tract carcinomas, and adverse fetal effects if cannabis is used in pregnancy.

The extremely high rates of cannabis use among drug misusers generally was demonstrated in a study of amphetamine, cocaine and heroin users both in and out of treatment (Robson & Bruce 1997). Of 581 users interviewed, 85% smoked cannabis, three-quarters of those having the drug every day. Budney et al. (1998) found that two-thirds of individuals presenting for treatment of opiate dependence smoked cannabis, nearly all of whom continued to do so during treatment with no apparent adverse effects on outcome. However, the cannabis users appeared to be a generally less stable group, in that they were more likely to report financial difficulties, be involved in drug dealing and engage in sharing needles, as well as being less likely to be married. The lack of any major influence of additional cannabis use on the broad beneficial outcomes of methadone maintenance treatment was also systematically demonstrated by Epstein and Preston (2003), although clearly this does not mean that cannabis problems should not be addressed in their own right.

In this book there have not been systematic examinations of the conceptual status and details of dependent states on the various drugs, but it is certainly worth noting that a condition comprising true dependence on cannabis is now recognized. In many ways the three cardinal features of dependence on a substance are tolerance, craving and withdrawal symptoms, and these have clearly been shown particularly in users presenting for treatment, for instance by Babor (2006) and Stephens et al. (2006). Also over 95% of the latter group's subjects had had unsuccessful attempts to quit or cut down, and usage continuing despite persistent or recurrent psychological or physical problems.

Treatment approaches found to be successful in cannabis problems have mainly been studied in primary users of the drug seeking help. They include motivational interviewing along standard lines (Miller & Rollnick 2002), cognitive-behavioural therapy (Stephens et al. 2000), and supportive-expressive psychotherapy, with the less personal treatments being with either individuals or groups (Stephens et al. 2006). Contingency management has also been tried, with this potentially being indicated for the secondary abuse of cannabis among opioid substitution patients. The comments of Budney et al. (2006) ring true when they observe that

In general, issues such as the relative harm of cannabis compared to other substances, the client's interest in abstaining from cannabis use, and the difficulty of abstaining from all substances versus just the primary one, must be given careful consideration when designing interventions to address secondary cannabis use.

The need to tailor cannabis treatments to a very diverse population of users has also been usefully considered by Steinberg et al. (2002).

Topic in brief – 10. Cannabis problems

- Clearly is often a 'gateway drug', although many use only this
- Persistent daily use is common, particularly in evenings to aid sleep
- Stronger forms appear to be producing more complications
- Long-term studies show association between early heavy use and subsequent mental illness, not solely attributable to related risk factors
- Treatment is mainly with various psychological approaches, with tailoring to circumstances necessary

---

Alcohol

Alcohol problems are the subject of many textbooks (e.g. Edwards et al. 2003), and only certain implications which are particularly relevant to the use of alcohol by drug misusers are considered here. The range of psychological adverse effects are well known, commonly including mood disturbances, anxiety as a withdrawal feature and, ultimately, cognitive impairment. Widespread physical effects include detectable liver damage as a relatively early feature in many cases and, although there is much individual variation in susceptibility to this damage, liver function tests are probably the single most useful objective indicator of heavy drinking, particularly the gamma glutamyl transferase result. This is reasonably specific to alcohol, although other common causes of a raised result include obesity, physical illnesses such as diabetes and many medications, while this test is especially useful in monitoring progress within the same individual, as the level changes quite rapidly with increases or decreases in alcohol intake. Increased red blood cell size on a full blood count is a more chronic feature, while the carbohydrate-deficient transferrin test is more specific to alcohol than the gamma glutamyl transferase but not used in routine practice. There are brief questionnaires to identify alcohol problems such as the Alcohol Use Disorders Identification Test (AUDIT) (Babor & Grant 1989), and even one which comprises a single question! This is: 'When was the last time you had more than eight drinks in one day?', or six drinks for women, with hazardous or harmful drinking suspected if the answer is within the past three months (Canagasaby & Vinson 2005). The classic description of a dependent state which can broadly be applied to any substance was first delineated in relation to alcohol (Edwards & Gross 1976), and in that way includes increased tolerance to alcohol, withdrawal symptoms and the relief of those symptoms by further drinking, subjective awareness of a compulsion to drink, and the stereotyping of a heavy-drinking routine.

The management of alcohol problems is barely less controversial than that of drug misuse, especially since a huge American study found hardly any significant relationships in attempts to match the various types of treatments to presenting problems (Mattson et al. 1998). In the past two decades or so the limited approach of giving advice on health risks and adhering to recommended safe levels of drinking, plus addressing the most immediate related problems, has been formalized in methods of 'brief intervention' (e.g. Fleming et al. 2002), while feedback of abnormal liver function results suspected to be due to alcohol should be done in practice and is often a useful motivating factor. Beyond that, various forms of counselling are made available, including by Alcoholics Anonymous, whose methods are readily embraced by a subgroup of alcohol misusers, although certainly not by all. The most useful medications (Lingford-Hughes et al. 2004) are chlordiazepoxide to alleviate alcohol withdrawal symptoms, disulfiram as a deterrent treatment in selected individuals who understand the risk of the potentially fatal disulfiram–ethanol reaction, and acamprosate, a more recently introduced medication which reduces desire for alcohol (Mann et al. 2004). The opioid antagonist naltrexone is used in several countries in the treatment of primary alcohol misusers, with the action of blocking receptors involved in the rewarding effects of alcohol, but this cannot of course be used in patients on methadone or other opioid substitutes. For a substantial minority of severely dependent drinkers detoxification in an inpatient or other residential setting is the only realistic option, and this makes it easier to administer parenteral vitamin B, which can be required to reduce the risk of complications such as Korsakoff's psychosis.

Most individuals who present with drug misuse have used alcohol at an earlier stage in their substance-using 'career', although a lack of liking for alcohol also seems relevant in some people starting drugs. The impression that significant use of alcohol at an early age is associated with various other behavioural and conduct problems and an increased likelihood of subsequent experimentation with drugs has been confirmed in studies (e.g. Federman et al. 1997), the implications therefore being similar to those of early use of cannabis. However, it would seem that as dependence on heroin in particular develops most individuals leave alcohol behind, in a way very aptly described by Lowe and Shewan (1999), so that a combined dependence is seen in only a minority of drug misusers in treatment (Gossop et al. 1998). In clinical practice with mainly opiate-dependent individuals there appears to be something of a bimodal distribution, at least in the early stages of treatment, whereby many will have little or no alcohol, a relatively small number will drink in moderation, and some will drink heavily combined with opiates and other drugs, clearly seeking definite intoxication. Ironically as treatment progresses and attempts are made by maintenance patients to stay off drugs, use of alcohol often increases, just as a switch to cocaine can occur in the way discussed earlier in this chapter. Also a period of drinking to excess seems even more common in drug-dependent individuals who do a full detoxification, with this actually being part of the rationale for continuing a stabilizing effect of methadone maintenance where this is achieved, as discussed in Chapter 1.

Overall, a factor which can be very relevant is parental history of alcoholism, with the additional complications related to this in addict offspring being demonstrated a long time ago by Kosten et al. (1985), including high levels of alcohol abuse again, and depression and personality disorder.

Drug misusers who also drink heavily can be very difficult to manage, with the standard treatments for alcohol misuse often seemingly compromised in this situation. As well as the process of tending to switch to drink in or after a monitored drug programme, when aspects of resocialization may be at work with patients 'getting back with normal friends who just have alcohol', it is also well-recognized that alcohol can boost the otherwise non-euphoriant effects of methadone. In cases where drinking seems to be partly to achieve this the ordinary treatment options for alcohol misuse are perhaps unlikely to be successful, and just as with patients who abuse benzodiazepines with methadone or buprenorphine there may seem more prospect of progress with a switch of maintenance agent, as discussed in Chapter 2. Certainly in large-scale examinations of reductions in substance use in opioid maintenance patients the results for alcohol tend to be among the worst, and indeed even when targetted counselling is undertaken in such users the effectiveness of that for alcohol seems to be less than that for drugs (Gossop et al. 2003, 2006).

Perhaps in general, the less obviously the alcohol is used to fill the euphoria 'gap' left by moving from street heroin to opioid substitution or full drug abstinence, the more fruitful the actual specific treatments for alcohol problems might be, but in all circumstances the many calls that there are for more attention to be paid to alcohol in ongoing treatment are surely correct. Testing for possible liver impairment effects is an obvious first step, and workers should definitely not be put off from doing this by the frequent difficulties in obtaining blood from intravenous users, or a belief that alcohol use is somehow not as relevant. Use should be made of specialist venepuncture services, and overall it has never been more necessary to address alcohol use in injecting addicts, given the increasing evidence of widespread hepatitis C infection and a particularly adverse effect of drinking on the prognosis of that condition (Rodger et al. 2000).

Case history

Sandra is in her early thirties, and was referred to our service when social services had concerns about neglect of her children and some violence in the home. She had actually been a patient of ours before, receiving methadone maintenance for a heroin problem dating back ten years, but in further allocating the cases within the city she had been directed to primary care management, because of her seemingly unproblematic progress.

When we received her back she was on a low and peculiar dose of methadone, and it transpired that she had recently been reducing this by 2 ml in the daily dosage every two weeks, at her own request. In the interview there was an obvious smell of alcohol, and assessment soon revealed that Sandra was drinking heavily every day, with her gamma glutamyl transferase coming back at several hundred international units per litre.

It did appear that a classic 'switch' to alcohol from drugs had occurred, and it also became apparent that Sandra had wanted to be seen to be reducing her methadone as well as giving clean urine samples, to look better for the social services. It was explained that this was very probably inadvisable, and that there was every chance that her drinking would simply increase with reductions in methadone, and titration back up to her previous maintenance dosage was advised. We felt it very important to explain our reasons for this to social services in the reports we provided, and it was accepted all round that by far the preferable situation would be for Sandra to be adhering to treatment medication only and avoiding any other substance abuse.

In the early stages of this latest period of treatment she was given strictly regulated supplies of chlordiazepoxide at home to help reduce her drinking, with it being explained that this would only be available if the evidence from her liver function tests did confirm that her drinking was less. In her renewed caseworking she was given specific advice on strategies to cut down alcohol use, with some related patient-friendly literature, and soon the benefits were obvious clinically. Her prescribing continued with acamprosate when she had established a period fully off alcohol, and her personal and home situations have greatly improved.

Nicotine

Drug misuse treatment services are often criticized for ignoring cigarette smoking, despite this being present in the overwhelming majority of their patients. In practice it can seem that few of the individuals presenting with problems from heroin and other illicit drugs envisage tackling smoking as well, but that is not always the case when the question is actually asked in studies (Sullivan & Covey 2002), and anyway the harms from nicotine are so severe and so well known that neglect of the issue is not justifiable. A body of public health evidence which lies outside the scope of this book shows the influence on smoking habits from broad controls such as bans in public places, while the provision of the respective kinds of services is separated in many countries by the treatment planners. In the UK the focus for smoking cessation programmes has been very clearly in primary care, with the helplines, literature and schemes such as national no-smoking days linked in with that setting, as well as funding for the medical treatments. We certainly share in common the issues of combatting high relapse rates, with a calculation from the time before widespread treatment in the USA that less than 10 per cent of nearly 20 million people who stopped smoking for at least one day remained abstinent one year later, although the more encouraging side was that a figure of the order of 40% gave up eventually (Fiore et al. 1994).

It is useful for clinicians in drug misuse services to know of the various approaches to smoking cessation, even though they may not be directly involved in deploying them. The treatments have been concisely reviewed by Aveyard and West (2007), and can be divided into four categories. Also, some reviews have particularly concentrated on smoking cessation in substance misusers (Sullivan & Covey 2002).

Brief therapies

These are a similar level of treatment to the minimal interventions used by primary care physicians to encourage patients to come off benzodiazepine tranquillizers, or moderate their alcohol intake. With the subject of smoking the advice on harms and any strategies for cutting down may well arise in the context of a consultation for a medical condition related to smoking, and has been described as '[one] extreme of smoking cessation interventions – opportunistic smoking cessation interventions by health care professionals (maximum reach, minimum effectiveness)' (McNeill et al. 2005). That is a paper which describes the national strategy for England, and illustrates the funding issues which pertain in smoking cessation, including that brief advice is not itself reimbursed but can be if there are wider measures attached to it in primary care such as training and service development. Brief advice alone has sometimes been the control treatment in studies of more specific behavioural interventions, with these usually finding added benefits for support for individuals, including by telephone, or in groups (Aveyard and West 2007).

Cognitive behaviour therapy

The cognitive-behavioural methods we are used to in drug misuse can be applied, especially in the management of cutting down rather than immediate cessation. As well as obvious measures such as increasing the 'inter-cigarette interval' and reducing amounts smoked at those intervals, other methods have attempted to weaken the positive reinforcement of smoking by allowing cigarettes at exact times rather than when desired. A common policy emphasis on abrupt quitting derives partly from findings such as gradual quitters being 40% less likely to succeed than those stopping abruptly in a general population study (West et al. 2001), but there may be some relevant differences between people who chose the two options (Hughes 2007).

Nicotine replacement treatment

Conceptually, this is familiar ground for drug workers, being the main use of a substitution treatment other than for opiates. There can be gums, lozenges and nasal sprays, with sometimes problems from these forms in gaining adequate dosing. The patch is probably the most reliable in this way, and there is a somewhat different principle, with the patch giving general nicotine replacement but the gum aimed at 'breakthrough' urges. This aspect is discussed by Aveyard and West (2007) along with the largest studies, and it is currently considered that nicotine replacement therapy almost doubles the success rates in cessation compared with placebo.

Some studies have added further interventions for patients receiving nicotine patches, including programmes on the internet. One large trial (Strecher et al. 2005) offered free web-based behavioural support to individuals who purchased a particular brand of patch, and found both general benefits, plus additional ones when the internet programme collected specific information from users and tailored advice to their needs.

Other medications

Antidepressants appear sometimes useful in aiding withdrawal attempts, rather as they can be in withdrawal from benzodiazepines or alcohol. There is some positive evidence for serotonin re-uptake inhibitors and nortriptyline, but the strongest is for bupropion, which in the UK at least is the only antidepressant licensed for use as a cessation aid. Success rates for this seem to be very similar to those with nicotine replacement, approximately doubling a smoker's chances (Hughes et al. 2007). The latest option is varenicline, which acts as a partial agonist on one of the nicotinic receptors.

This, bupropion and nicotine replacement can all be first-line choices, with previous experience of the patient and their own views very important, given that smoking is a form of substance dependence which tends to be overcome mainly through individuals' own efforts.

Providing clinical services
Community drug services

Introduction

This book is written from the perspective of working within multidisciplinary community-based treatment services for drug misusers. In the UK these are not a minority type of service subsumed under more institutionalized treatment, but rather they represent the main model of treatment delivery in this speciality in most areas. They are primarily clinical, with most of the work comprising counselling of various kinds for the drug misusers who have been referred, along with medical input and the provision of pharmacological treatments. The teams are part of the National Health Service, with funding often coming jointly from health and social services. Typically most workers are community psychiatric nurses or social workers, with much overlap in the type of casework undertaken. The extent to which teams are involved in nonclinical projects, such as needle exchange schemes, outreach, drug information or relatives' groups, depends largely on the availability of other services, particularly from the nonstatutory sector, and carving out a suitable role for a clinical community drug service is an important challenge. Many lessons have been learnt as such services have emerged from the shadow of the previously dominant drug dependence units (DDUs), as a brief history of this process of development will illustrate.

Of course as community teams have become established there has been branching out into various more specialized areas of work, for instance in projects to do with recently released prisoners, individuals on court orders, pregnant addicts, etc., and such schemes will not themselves be described as some are very specific to the UK. In Chapter 8, however, there will be examination of the types of work undertaken with the range of special patient groups.

Historical development

The formation of nonmedical multidisciplinary community drug teams (CDTs) was originally recommended in a highly influential report of the Advisory Council on the Misuse of Drugs, the UK's central advisory body which is set up by statute (Advisory Council on the Misuse of Drugs 1982). Among a series of reports, this one laid down the desirable structure of treatment and rehabilitation services for drug misusers within the country, and it was envisaged that each health district, with populations of around a quarter of a million people, would have such a drug team. Their main role was seen not so much as direct provision of clinical treatment to limited numbers of users, but the facilitation of treatment and rehabilitation by a wider network of professionals. This nonmedical team would therefore have links with a local consultant psychiatrist in drug misuse and their junior doctors, and primary care physicians, as well as with nonstatutory drug agencies, probation, social services and other organizations in contact with drug users. The CDT had premises in a community location, preferably in a town centre, and joint treatment for a client would usually comprise counselling at the CDT base plus appointments at the local consultant's outpatient clinic, or their own primary care physician's office. Over and above these local clinical services each of the regions, which could comprise 10–20 health districts, would have a more specialized drug misuse service with full-time consultants, bigger medical and multidisciplinary teams and additional facilities such as an inpatient unit. Such services were expected to generally treat the more difficult cases, and were typically based where there had previously been the substantial DDUs.

These Advisory Council on the Misuse of Drugs recommendations can be seen as very formative in the deinstitutionalization of drug misuse treatment in the UK, as previously the DDUs had overseen the treatment of most of the known addicts in their areas, with the disadvantages of long-distance travelling for patients and lack of involvement of generic services. As rates of drug misuse generally increased, with clinical treatments clearly indicated for a substantial proportion of the new heroin users, it was recognized that general practitioners and a wide range of other doctors and associated clinicians would need to be involved. These principles were reinforced still further a few years later as drug misusers became implicated in the HIV epidemic, when there was a consequent emphasis on widespread low-threshold treatment (Advisory Council on the Misuse of Drugs 1988, 1989). Throughout the 1980s many posts were therefore created to form the new CDTs, who were required to have a role in training as well as the provision and facilitation of treatment.

The model of community drug services has endured, with important changes of emphasis which are detailed below. As time has progressed they have become even more the focus of treatment for most areas, since changes in the National Health Service have meant that the conventional regional and district structure in administration and provision has largely been dismantled. With decentralization and some scaling down of regional services, most districts covering populations of a quarter to half a million are needing to become more self-sufficient in drug misuse treatment. The largest services which previously operated on a regional basis are needing to re-evaluate their role, concentrating for instance on newer methods of inpatient opiate detoxification or on providing outpatient prescribing services for individuals who require nonstandard medication regimes.

The focus here is on treatment within community drug services, as these have evolved in the face of changing demands.

Changes in emphasis

The practicalities of working in CDTs, as services stood at the time, were described by Strang et al. (1992). The main aspects are summarized in Table 5.1.

The multidisciplinary composition of teams was seen as fundamental to this service model. Strang et al. (1992) noted that this related strongly to the liaison element of the work so that, for instance, links with social services would be more effectively forged if the approach came from a social worker in a CDT. As CDTs took on more direct treatment the benefits had more to do with skill mix for their own clinical work, and were perhaps more arguable. Most posts were for community psychiatric nurses and social workers, with some unqualified drug workers who might be ex-users. Having workers from different disciplines with their own 'line managers' could pose problems for overall team management, and often there was a coordinator post to include that role.

Table 5.1 The work of community drug teams

Composition of teams
Community psychiatric nurses, social workers, other drug counsellors, management, administration, plus medical input
Catchment area
Local, defined
Clinical treatment
Triage
Facilitation of treatment by others
Direct treatment of medium-severity cases
General roles
Counselling
Advice and information
Telephone help-line
Drop-in service
Needle exchange
Outreach
General medical services

Based on Strang et al. (1992)

A complement of four full-time and two part-time workers, including a secretary and a coordinator, was considered about average at that time, which now seems very small given the expansions which have occurred! The catchment area would be absolutely defined, with the advantage that the team would get to know their local area and its services well, and make the links with other agencies in the community. As in other specialities in psychiatry, the community ethos of treatment relates to links of this kind, as well as to location of services and an emphasis on visits to home and other settings.

Initially, medical treatment was seen as an aspect which was provided elsewhere, through liaison as indicated above. Gradually the nonmedical and medical elements of treatment have become more integrated, to the extent that the term 'CDT' is somewhat outdated as describing nonmedical personnel only. Partly this integration has been desired, with consultants for instance preferring to do their clinics for drug misusers at CDT premises, rather than have patients brought to them by workers. As well as the benefits of convenience for the patient and better communication between doctor and team, this gets away from the perception of a worker acting as a separate advocate for a drug user in their dealings with the doctor. Also, however, prescribing in particular has had to move 'in-house' as drug services acknowledged that they needed to carry out direct treatment in a large proportion of cases. The original CDT concept implied a kind of 'triage' system, in which drug users with routine prescription needs could be treated by their own primary care physicians with guidance, some especially problematic individuals might need referral to a regional centre, and only a limited number would require all aspects of management to be from the drug service. Assessing nearly a decade of the setting-up and operating of CDTs, Strang et al. (1992) observed that '[because] the extent of collaboration from generic colleagues (especially general practitioners) has been poor... an unplanned abandonment of the original consultancy role for the CDT is widely evident, as CDT workers have become more actively involved in the delivery of care'. Offering in-house prescribing might be considered to compound the difficulty of encouraging generic services to become involved with treating drug misusers, but it simply became a necessary pragmatic development. At a time when the importance of contact with services was being emphasized because of HIV, drug teams with medical services were found to see six times as many heroin users, three times as many amphetamine users, and five times as many injecting drug misusers overall, as comparable teams without such input (Strang et al. 1991).

In mentioning the possible general roles for a CDT as listed in Table 5.1, Strang et al. (1992) suggested that all except drug counselling and the provision of advice and information lay outside the original brief (Advisory Council on the Misuse of Drugs 1982). Drug counselling is of course central to the work of nonmedical members of drug treatment services, and is considered further below. Services inevitably feel the need to give advice to drug users and relatives contacting them in their area, but use can also be made of the various national telephone helplines and drug information outlets. The division of activities between a clinical service and any local 'street agencies' run by nonstatutory organizations for drug users is important to establish, and the latter routinely provide much information and contact telephone numbers on a drop-in basis. There are inevitable areas of overlap, but it is generally more appropriate for informal contacts, nonspecific support and needle exchange to also be at the street agency. The difficulties of reconciling injecting equipment provision with clinical sessions, in which some users may not fully acknowledge their additional drug use, have been recognized ever since harm-reduction measures were introduced, and even where both kinds of assistance are provided from the same service there needs to be a degree of separation.

Outreach services in drug misuse (Grund et al. 1992) may include distributing injecting equipment, informal health promotion, efforts to recruit younger heroin users into treatment, or initiatives related to other drugs, such as advising on safer use of stimulants in nightclub attenders. Once again, in areas where there is a street drug agency this work is increasingly seen as being mainly in their province, for a number of reasons. Some of these are practical, relating to unusual working hours and conditions, while others are to do with the various skills required for different kinds of work, and the need to orient professional staff more to clinical treatment. In the current employment and medico-legal climates there are potential problems in having health service staff involved in the more inventive fringes of drug outreach work, just as there can be pitfalls the other way round in, for instance, having ex-users advising on prescribed treatments.

There are precedents for both statutory and nonstatutory services offering general health care sessions for drug misusers who do not contact general practitioners. Morrison and Ruben (1995) described such a scheme, in which a general practitioner provided four sessions a week at a centre aimed at HIV-preventive activities. The authors pointed out that not only did many drug users fail to access direct treatment for drug misuse or ordinary health care services from primary care physicians, but many more were not even registered with a doctor. Their service was also aimed at prostitutes, and concentrated on HIV and hepatitis testing, hepatitis B vaccination, sexually transmitted infection screening and contraception. It had long been recognized that drug services tend not to be active enough in pursuing hepatitis B vaccination (Farrell et al. 1990), with a study of drug misusers in police custody finding that only 10% were aware of its availability, despite nearly 50% being in contact with treatment services (Payne-James et al. 1994).

Much of the ethos of community drug treatment as it has developed has been firmly grounded in 'harm-reduction' policies. There is frequent debate as to exactly what such principles entail, and even how appropriate they are in countries at different stages of development. Those interested in the philosophy are referred to a paper by AL Ball (2007) from the department of HIV/Aids at the World Health Organization, which clearly still sees avoidance of HIV as one of the key aims of this policy agenda. A short commentary on that article succinctly sums up the areas of importance in drug service provision, as follows:

providing clean injecting equipment to injecting drug users, agonist maintenance treatment for opioid dependence, education about blood-borne virus risk behaviour and ways of reducing it, HIV testing and counselling, and access to antiretroviral therapy and more effective treatments for hepatitis C virus to [drug users]. If better evidence becomes available, one might add to the list supervised injecting facilities in settings with high rates of high-risk street injecting.

(Hall 2007)

Some further developments

As already indicated, this chapter is a broad-brush picture of community services, which it is hoped will be of interest in areas and countries with other types of provision. The book in general concentrates on actual clinical treatment, and the special aspects of treatment in particular patient groups are discussed in the final chapter. Keeping matters very general, there have been three further significant trends in the development of community drug services in the UK.

The first is the major growth of prescribing services and other medical provision to drug misusers by general practitioners, in addition to the services which are psychiatrically based, and primary care treatment is discussed shortly. This does not mean that there have been great changes in the willingness of primary care physicians to routinely provide treatment from their own premises or for their own patients, but rather many doctors have gone into drug misuse full-time as 'primary care specialists'. Broadly speaking, services led by these doctors are not as multidisciplinary as the kinds of services described above where the prescribing and other medical sessions are done by psychiatrists, and the skill mix in attached staff is also somewhat different, with perhaps more from nonstatutory agencies and fewer community psychiatric nurses. When both kinds of services exist in a district there is a natural tendency in service organization, or 'purchasing', for the psychiatric services to be asked to concentrate on so-called 'dual diagnosis' work, a subject discussed by many observers (Abou-Saleh 2007, Drake et al. 2007), and elsewhere in this book. Of course this would be too narrow a focus in itself, as substance misuse has simply been mainly a speciality of psychiatry since the current forms of illicit drug use started, and so the standard psychiatrically based services have developed expertise across the range of types of cases, and still have that.

A second change has been a great emphasis on treatment aimed at crime reduction, with expansion of services in the UK and elsewhere which can really be seen as another 'wave', following the major one in the 1990s after the recognition of the HIV threat (Advisory Council on the Misuse of Drugs 1989). Many schemes have been set up to enable 'diversion' from some forms of sentencing for addicts who are willing to undergo treatment for drug problems, usually tied to more intensive monitoring than is routine in ordinary modern clinical treatment (Ryder et al. 2001).

Finally, although clearly this summary is not comprehensive, there has been yet another big change as there have been more calls for services to benefit users of non-opiate drugs, as well as the opiate addicts in substitution treatment, with the great rise in cocaine problems being prominent in this way (Gossop et al. 2002a). As has been discussed in chapter 4, the management of non-opiate misuse and dependence is much less clinical than services have been used to with opiate addicts, and so this work has been spread across more types of services, including the nonstatutory. These kinds of agencies have been able to respond positively to this trend, with development beyond needle exchanges, information provision and drop-in services to include for instance group counselling and advice for crack users, and acupuncture and complementary therapies.

Organization within teams

Mention is made here of some features within general community team working which we have found beneficial in our own services.

- Sectorization

  Each of the workers within a core team primarily covers one geographical sector, based on local government boundaries. The advantages of sectorization are well recognized, and include not only the worker becoming familiar with local services, personnel and drug scenes, but also the local users getting to know the worker. Often referrals are enabled in this way, and sometimes the worker will already know of a newly presenting individual through other contacts, which helps in general assessment. There is also a back-up system, in which one other worker takes a proportion of referrals from the area and makes the contacts to a lesser degree, which is useful at times such as holiday cover or periods when additional input is required.

- Any referral source, including self-referral

  In one of our services referrals can be taken from any source, including primary care, probation, social services or other agencies, or individuals may self-refer. Self-referral is actually the most frequent route, which is probably a good indicator of the general level of satisfaction with the service. This wider policy, as opposed to our practice in the main city of accepting mainly from primary care physicians and having no self-presentations, is made possible by the reasonably high staffing level and an absence of a large city concentration of opiate users.

- Duty worker system

  Each weekday afternoon one of the workers is available to see self-referrals or other individuals presenting, and to give telephone advice to anyone who requires it. Such contacts need to be reasonably brief and, in the case of new referrals, usually initial details are taken so that a worker can be allocated to the individual at the weekly team meeting. In some situations where an urgent response is indicated, such as starting naltrexone in an individual presenting drug-free (see Chapter 3), this is arranged after appropriate testing. Relevant preliminary advice is given in all newly presenting cases, including written information where possible. For other contacts, the duty worker system is designed to reduce the frustration for individuals of having nobody available to answer queries, including when a client's own worker may be out doing community visits.

- Emphasis on home and community visits
  With a large geographical area it is considered unreasonable to expect clients to always attend the service base. They need to do so for the set medical clinic sessions, but many appointments with the drug workers are either at home or at other community offices. Once again the advantages of home visits are well known, including seeing a client's circumstances and talking to relatives or partners, while we also do not expect individuals undergoing quick detoxifications to travel. The sectorization of the service makes for increased efficiency of a community policy, in terms of travelling time and costs.

- Active keyworking
  The keyworker role is considered very important with all clients of the services. Once a worker is allocated to a case, they take the main treatment decisions, with supervision provided and in collaboration with the prescribing doctor. In normal circumstances such decisions are not over-ridden in duty worker contacts, and clients are made aware of this. Because the system is adhered to consistently there are relatively few attempts to problematically exploit it, and in general this approach is well accepted.

  The keyworker role is a very active one with, for instance, much support and encouragement provided to young users who wish to detoxify. In established opioid maintenance patients, medical appointments may occur only two to three times per year, with all the intervening contacts with the keyworker. Here the agenda is conspicuously not to alter the maintenance polices, but to assist and advise regarding various important additional aspects, ranging from social problems to engagement with general medical care. In all clients for whom treatment is underway or planned, regular contact is strongly encouraged.

  Much of the work of ours and other community drug services comes into the category of drug counselling, and this will now be examined in a little more detail.

Drug counselling

This term potentially includes a wide range of approaches, from informal support to specific techniques such as motivational interviewing (Noonan & Moyers 1997), and the particular methods adopted in rehabilitation centres or 12-step programmes. In clinical services in the UK and elsewhere, a concept of drug counselling is prevalent which includes providing various types of practical advice in different situations, but also incorporates elements which are relatively targeted in aiming at behavioural change; in Chapter 3 we discussed such approaches in relation to detoxification and relapse prevention. This kind of work is fundamental to drug services as, to varying degrees, counselling is indicated for virtually all individuals who present. Table 5.2 indicates some of the main elements of drug counselling, which are not highly specialized in nature, but may be useful measures to adopt with or without the application of more specific clinical treatments. Particularly in forms of drug misuse for which no pharmacological treatments are indicated, such approaches may be the most useful input in helping an individual reduce harmful behaviours and cut down or stop drug-taking.

As already discussed, harm reduction is in itself a large subject, but the behaviour change measures which should be adopted by individuals can readily be covered in counselling. Sexual risk-taking behaviour is notoriously more difficult to change than behaviours relating to drugs, and both aspects must be addressed. Health advice may be concerned with specific adverse effects of drugs, side-effects of medication, general aspects

Table 5.2 Elements of general drug counselling

Harm-reduction advice – drugs, sex

Health advice

Changing drug-taking behaviours

Changing lifestyle

Dealing with cravings, stress

Problem-solving

Social skills

Psychological aspects – self-esteem, anxiety and depression

such as nutrition, or testing, vaccination and treatment for infectious complications. Beyond basic harm-reduction advice, individuals can be counselled more specifically regarding tactics for reducing drug usage, changing route and modifying drug-taking in various ways. There may be related lifestyle changes to consider, to do with networks of friends, social activities or more major changes such as moving area. Dealing with craving overlaps with this, for which techniques range from those based on distraction, to specific cognitive-behavioural training on responding to cues (Pollack et al. 2002).

There are further areas in which the counselling becomes somewhat more specialized, and psychological, in nature, relating to difficulties which are common in drug misusers. It may be necessary to advise on methods of coping with stress, to enhance problem-solving or social skills, or to address significant problems of low self-esteem, anxiety or depression. With the casework of drug team members generally being very similar this may fall to most types of worker, but clearly community psychiatric nurses and psychologists are particularly well placed to administer counselling of this kind.

Importantly, the counselling techniques as deployed in standard form may need significant modifications for individuals with additional psychiatric illness, and given the increasing emphasis on this population within psychiatrically based drug services there is much discussion of this aspect in Chapter 7.

Topic in brief – 11. Providing drug counselling

- Should usually be integral in each case, rather than just a possible 'add-on' to medication
- A keyworker model, with attention to practical and lifestyle issues, plus behaviourally based advice on reducing drug use is widely applicable
- Typically includes elements of cognitive-behavioural therapy, e.g. in dealing with cravings and trigger situations, and motivational interviewing
- Is preferably from the same service as the prescribing, to enable easy joint working and avoid the need for 'lobbying'

6

Providing clinical services
Treatment of drug misuse in primary care

Introduction

Liasion with primary care physicians is a fundamental tenet of community psychiatry, with the aim of joint treatment between community team members and the doctors, and this certainly applies to drug treatment services in many countries. It is often pointed out that the whole situation of there being waiting lists for methadone and other treatments from some specialist services would be solved if each primary care physician treated the drug users on his or her patient list, but in reality this amount of 'spreading around' does not happen. Although by definition I and my direct colleagues are not actually involved in the provision of primary care treatment, it is fairly easy to identify from the literature the obstacles which exist to widespread treatment, and much effort has been put into overcoming these in our own city of Sheffield. The various moves to try and encourage treatment have aroused strong emotions, so that when I very first took up post in Sheffield I noticed that the front cover of a local general practice newsletter was exhorting members to 'man the barricades' against what seemed to me like an over-enthusiastic scheme that was being proposed. A decade and a half later, Sheffield resembles many other UK cities in having only limited direct involvement of general practitioners actually in primary care in treating addicts, in terms of numbers of addicts on approved treatments per practice, and instead much of the prescribing being done from a primary care specialist service, i.e. led by general practitioners who have gone into drug misuse full-time (Keen et al. 2003).

Probably the most important aspects in briefly reviewing primary care treatment are the effectiveness of provision, and the differences in treatment methods which can occur because of the nature of the setting, and these will be examined. This chapter mainly adopts the perspective of treatment in the UK, where there are no major administrative restrictions on managing drug misusers in primary care, and therefore much experience to draw on.

Levels of interest

A point which often seems to be ignored in the many surveys of 'attitudes' of primary care physicians towards drug misusers is that our speciality of substance misuse is only one of hundreds which the doctors have to deal with, in terms of presenting problems, treatment guidelines, shared care with the relevant specialist services etc. It is completely unsurprising that the levels of involvement of different doctors and practices are going to vary widely, and some of the surveys undertaken do validly pick up on the issue of whether primary care physicians even consider that drug misuse should be managed in their setting. I have already indicated that feelings can run high, not just because of personal views but because the realists among doctors accept that the nature of primary care, with limited appointment times, no special facilities and less security than in the specialist centres, renders it vulnerable to exploitation by the proportion of active drug misusers so inclined. The undoubtedly mixed picture which emerges was well illustrated in a national survey of general practitioners in Scotland by Matheson et al. (2003), which found 60% of responding primary care physicians to be treating drug users, with 52% providing methadone. However, in the section on attitudes and beliefs, nearly half of doctors agreed or strongly agreed with the statements 'prescribing a controlled drug to drug misusers is not part of a GP's professional remit' and 'drug misusers in my practice would endanger staff safety', and almost as many with 'drug misusers visiting my practice would discourage other patients'.

An informal categorization of levels of interest of primary care physicians in treating drug misusers is presented in Box 6.1. This does not include full-time primary care specialists, but there has been formalization in the UK of 'general practitioners with special interests', or GPSIs, with this model having been reviewed by Gerada and Limber (2003). The definition of a GPSI is 'a GP with appropriate experience who is able to independently deliver a specialist service, working in a clinical area outside the normal remit of general practice care ... [they work] in an appropriate venue within a defined quality framework and [are] able to accept referrals from GPs and other professional colleagues'. A specific issue for the UK, but with parallels elsewhere, is the extent to which treatment of opiate dependence falls within one of the main contracts of employment, the General Medical Services contract (Felice & Kouimtsidis 2008), while it has also been found that primary care physicians attracted to the special training in this subject tend to anyway be those with positive attitudes towards the patient group (Strang et al. 2007a). There has probably been an overall trend to not concentrate extensive resources on those doctors unsympathetic to drug misusers (i.e. level four in the description here), although those interested in 'engaging the reluctant general practitioner' are referred to a systematic study of 'change-orientated reflective listening' (Strang et al. 2004), i.e. as the paper indicates, a kind of motivational interviewing for staff!

The principle of the more straightforward and routine cases being managed in primary care, with more difficult problems being referred to specialists, whether themselves general practitioners or the specialist psychiatrists, is inherent in many health care systems and of course not just in drug misuse. Even so, Brownell and Naik (2003) found in a survey

---

Box 6.1. Levels of interest of primary care physicians in treating drug misusers

Level 1
Substantially involved, e.g. working in a drug misuse service or providing special clinics in primary care. Particularly interested in this patient group.

Level 2
More limited involvement, e.g. offering treatment to a small number in conjunction with a drug service. No major objections, provided situation can be contained.

Level 3
Not currently offering treatment but would do so if additional training and support were made available.

Level 4
Opposed to treatment taking place in primary care, perhaps vehemently. Probably also reluctant to have drug misusers as patients for general medical care. May be a personal opinion or a practice policy.

regarding whether general practitioners were providing four government-defined 'key services' for drug misusers that 'there is a huge gap between current provision and government expectations, which may be unrealistic'. They found that half of the doctors who had read the government guidelines on treatment provision were not willing to change their practice, although Strang et al. (2007b) demonstrated a stronger influence of prescribing guidelines on the treatment from general practitioners with methadone and buprenorphine in England, with subsequently higher doses of methadone, more frequent dispensing and supervised consumption, and less use of methadone tablets.

Mention was made in the sections in earlier chapters discussing buprenorphine that in some countries this drug is more associated with treatment in primary care, and methadone within specialist services. This has been both because of the perceived greater safety of buprenorphine, including when there is take-home dispensing rather than supervised consumption at a treatment centre, and also to do with patient populations, i.e. that there may be a more 'middle-class' population of opiate-dependent individuals who are prepared to see their own primary care physician but would not attend a methadone service. In France there was some concern that the use of buprenorphine in primary care might be too lax in terms of required attendance and urine sampling to produce strong benefits in treatment, but where similar policies to those in specialist centres have been adopted very comparable results across settings have been demonstrated, there and elsewhere (Vignau & Brunelle 1998, Ortner et al. 2004).

Effectiveness

There are now a large number of studies demonstrating similar effectiveness of methadone and/or buprenorphine prescribing within primary care and other services. Broadly this is to be expected, since as discussed in Chapter 1 it is virtually impossible to provide opioid maintenance treatment in any systematic way without achieving routine reductions in opiate use, injecting, crime, family problems, etc. In some ways a classic example of this kind of demonstration was provided by Keen et al. (2003), who examined outcomes of methadone maintenance at one year in an open study and found reduced heroin use, convictions and cautions, HIV risk-taking behaviours and problems of social functioning and health. This study was in our own city of Sheffield, and indeed illustrates a modern dilemma about the provision of treatment in different settings. The very title of the paper poses the question whether 'methadone maintenance treatment based on the new national guidelines work(s) in a primary care setting?', but actually the setting is itself a specialist service in its own premises, headed by doctors who have given up general practice to go into drug misuse treatment full-time. Whether this actually constitutes primary care has been the subject of much local debate, which I am sure is reflected in other places!

A wide range of studies of methadone and buprenorphine maintenance were included in a review in a general practice journal by Simoens et al. (2005), although most of the studies had been in other specialist clinics. Similar results between such studies and the trials of treatment in primary care were found, although it was noted that for 'office practice' some criteria for clinical stability were required. The authors concluded 'that evidence is emerging in favour of primary care treatment with methadone and buprenorphine. However, this is perhaps only feasible for subjects who meet criteria of sufficient clinical stability. Moreover, appropriate training of primary care physicians is essential'. In general it seems that the strongest evidence in opioid substitution comes from shared care schemes where security measures are implemented, for instance daily supervised consumption of methadone as in a study of one-year follow-up of opiate injectors treated in a liaison scheme in Glasgow (Hutchinson et al. 2000). The results were based on self-reports from the users, but in this way it appeared that individuals who had remained on methadone for the whole year had reduced daily injecting from 78% to 2% and daily drugs spend from £50 to £4, with also marked reductions in crime.

Where treatment is provided in outright primary care, rather than a secondary service run by doctors with a primary care background, a common model is to have a liaison worker from the specialist community drug service also see the cases. Typically the drug worker sees the user at the practice premises, either at the same time as the primary care physician or in effect doing a 'clinic' there at intervals, and takes care of drug testing as well as any relevant counselling. He or she then has liaison discussions with the doctor about the prescribing aspects, with this often being a chance to give advice on implementing daily supervised consumption at a community pharmacy, at least at the early stages of treatment. A form of service delivery of this kind found to be very effective has been to offer primary care physicians practice-based review for clients developing chaotic drug use, assistance with the transfer of patients in a specialist team into shared care, and continuing support and training on drug-related issues (Dey et al. 2002).

Some characteristics of primary care treatment

Among all the studies, largely surveys, of primary care physicians' attitudes towards drug misusers and preparedness to provide treatment, relatively little attention is paid to the treatment of actual physical conditions, including the various ones relating to injecting. A concern undoubtedly exists that if the doctors are unsympathetic to drug misusers anyway then even general medical care will be denied, with either the drug user not feeling that their doctor is 'helpful' and therefore not attending, or opportunites being taken by the practice to remove drug users from the list because of, for instance, unreliability with appointments or perhaps aggressive outbursts. It would seem, however, that where drug misusers do engage with their primary care physician the investigation and management of complicating physical problems could be better than that provided in the psychiatric clinics, and that does seem to be the view of many observers (e.g. Carnwath et al. 2000). That paper is an account of a substantial shared care scheme in the Manchester area in the UK, with the authors themselves having much experience in primary care. Based on that experience they make the point that 'Any general practitioner trained in recent decades will confirm that the training focuses on a patient-centred approach where the consultation serves as the medium for establishing patient problems and concerns, and agreeing a management [says problem, presumably plan] in the light of patient expectations'. They are actually making the point that it is surprising that some primary care physicians in deprived areas of large cities can actually decide not to treat drug misusers, even though it is going to be one of the most common conditions among young people in those places, but the consideration about the patient-centred approach is interesting on another level also, as follows.

Although there have not been examinations of the link between such a philosophy and the policies and treatment practices adopted, it is likely that an approach which is driven by the patient's preferences and seeks to avoid any disagreement or confrontation will be associated with practices which could be popular, but also less secure than advised. Certainly the extent of the departure from the original model of methadone maintenance

Table 6.1 Treatment in specialist services and primary care

Specialist services	
Advantages	**Disadvantages**
Detailed background knowledge of treatments	Stigma
Services specifically oriented to patient group	Travelling
Easier to apply required security measures	Association of many users together may be problematic
Efficiency from managing many similar cases	Sometimes waiting lists for maintenance
Primary care	
Advantages	**Disadvantages**
Personalized service, local	Setting more readily exploited by drug misusers
Less stigma	Brief appointments allow for prescribing medication but not for more challenging aspects
More expertise in investigating and managing physical conditions	May be pressure to act with inadequate information
Widespread involvement can reduce waits for treatment	Involvement when other doctors are not can lead to excessive demand

clinics is starkly illustrated in the survey by Matheson et al. (2003) referred to above, in which 38% of general practitioners providing treatment said that they 'hardly ever' or 'never' carried out urine testing, and 45% were supplying maintenance benzodiazepines. The latter subject has been discussed at length elsewhere in this book, including referring to an exceptionally high prevalence of benzodiazepine misuse by addicts in Scotland where that survey was carried out, and perhaps benzodiazepines were being given sometimes as a response to a perceived dependence problem. The issue, however, is a potentially troublesome one right across primary care services, with a study from Australia finding that heroin addicts had greatly increased rates of presentation to general practitioners and receipt of benzodiazepines than would be normal for non-drug patients (Darke et al. 2003). Some researchers have taken the view that if it is wished to know what prescribing practices are occurring, then the best place to look is the pharmacies where prescriptions are dispensed as per instructions, rather than asking doctors in surveys what they do. A major such study was carried out in the UK by Strang et al. (2007b), who compared the frequency of methadone or buprenorphine dispensing on prescriptions issued by drug dependency clinic specialists, general practitioners and doctors in private practice. For methadone, clinic prescriptions were most likely to be for daily dispensing, with a lower proportion for this in general practice and a much lower proportion in private practice, which could indicate the extent to which patients' requests for less frequent collection are agreed to. Of course in many areas primary care physicians would at least in theory have the more straightforward patients who could perhaps have been drug-free and therefore more suitable for take-home medication, but the possibilities come full circle when it is recalled that the trend is for less testing in primary care and so drug use might not be detected! The value therefore of such large-scale comparisons is limited in one way, and clinicians in their own areas will tend to know the philosophy of different services and doctors.

To conclude, some general advantages and disadvantages of specialist and primary care settings can be indicated, although again much variation in individual services will occur.

Topic in brief – 12. Characteristics of primary care management of opiate addicts

- Advisory guidelines have only limited impact, with recommended policies not necessarily implemented
- Much of the involvement of primary care physicians is from a subgroup especially interested in the subject, sometimes in 'primary care specialist' services
- Liaison work from drug services can effectively increase and complement primary care treatment
- Substitute prescribing tends to be on a more 'take-home' basis and with less drug testing than in specialist services

Providing clinical services
Dual diagnosis – drug misuse and psychiatric disorder

Introduction

One of the reasons why drug misuse is managed substantially as a psychiatric speciality is that it is strongly associated with various pervasive and clinically important psychiatric conditions. Studies have examined the relationship both ways round – that is, investigating rates of mental disorders in drug misusers, or the extent of drug misuse in mentally ill populations, and some of these are discussed here. In practice, clinicians must be skilled in recognizing personality disorder (often as a continuation of adolescent conduct disorder), depression and anxiety states, all of which are extremely common and need to be distinguished from the effects of drug misuse itself. Personality disorder is particularly important, as it is often the main cause of abnormal mood in drug misusers and it exerts strong negative effects on many aspects of management; the first part of the chapter focuses on this, the other main associated conditions and also the difficult area of drug-induced psychosis. The rest of the chapter is then given over to a discussion from the other perspective, of substance misuse problems in those with severe mental illness, as the rising rates of such problems are currently posing great difficulties in the provision of general psychiatric treatment in the community.

The management of those with schizophrenia and other psychotic conditions who misuse drugs is highly problematic, partly because such individuals do not comply well with conventional addiction treatment approaches, and a literature is emerging which is largely on ultra-specialist services for that group. A wider difficulty is that the drugs involved are often not opiates, and so even if engagement is encouraged, there are few specific clinical treatments which can be applied. If only because of the particular vulnerability of those with severe mental illness, however, and the propensity of various drugs to worsen psychosis, such users need to be accorded some priority in services, especially those which are psychiatrically based. The case for ultra-specialist services for this group is arguable, but some fundamental treatment principles which have been identified from such services are examined here, and appear to have good general applicability. In many areas there is no special service provision, beyond perhaps having identified dual diagnosis workers, and much reliance needs to be placed on good liaison and joint working between general psychiatric and drug misuse teams.

Table 7.1 lists the main additional psychiatric disorders encountered in drug misusers, in approximate ranking. In general, psychosis is found to be much rarer than the conditions at the top of the list, certainly single figure percentage prevalence rates in most studies, but there are very particular implications which will be discussed. In terms of overall prevalence of psychiatric conditions in drug misusers, many studies of a decade or so ago found very

Table 7.1 Most common psychiatric disorders in studies of drug misusers

Personality disorder
Other substance misuse
Depression
Anxiety
Psychosexual dysfunction
Psychotic disorders

high occurrence, for instance from 60 to 90% (Musselman & Kell 1995, Kokkevi et al. 1998, Mason et al. 1998), but these are probably too high to be truly representative since the studies were of clinical samples in specialized (sometimes psychiatric) treatment settings. In fact it could be argued that even studies that are purely of opiate-dependent individuals will find unduly high rates, as possibly the more disordered individuals progress to the most addictive form of drug use, and so there has also been interest in household surveys. Of these, in the Epidemiologic Catchment Area (ECA) study of over 20 000 people seen by lay interviewers in the USA (Regier et al. 1990), the lifetime prevalence of some additional psychiatric condition in individuals with diagnosable substance abuse or dependence was 53%, while in the UK psychiatric disorder was found with a standardized clinical rating instrument to be present in 22% of nicotine-dependent individuals, 30% of alcohol-dependent and 45% of drug-dependent, as against 12% of the non-dependent population (Farrell et al. 2001).

A careful and large clinical investigation across three UK cities in effect bridged this gap between service statistics and general population findings, by surveying over 2500 community mental health team patients and 1600 substance misuse service attenders to investigate the reciprocal conditions, with almost complete compliance with the survey (Weaver et al. 2003). In individuals receiving treatment for drug misuse there were prevalence rates of 68% for depression and/or anxiety, 8% for non-substance-induced psychotic disorders and 37% for personality disorders (Bowden-Jones et al. 2004), with this last figure actually being higher for alcohol cases, which is an unusual finding. For some figures 'the other way round', in that study 31% of the community mental health team sample had current illicit drug use, with all these rates of disorders coming from sub-samples of interviewed cases. In the ECA study the lifetime prevalence of substance misuse in the mentally ill was 29%, this rising to 47% in those with schizophrenia.

Mental disorders in drug misusers

Looking at the listing of disorders found in drug misusers, it can readily be seen that a very common issue must be to satisfactorily separate the true conditions themselves from effects of either the activity of drug misuse, effects and withdrawal effects of drugs (depression as withdrawal from stimulants, anxiety from sedatives) and even side-effects of medications (e.g. psychosexual dysfunction). This will be particularly examined in the sections which follow on personality disorder and on depression, while in the case of anxiety disorders it is usually very strongly recommended to avoid benzodiazepines in drug misusers (but also see the section on prescribing these in Chapter 2). When it is felt that psychological counselling is indicated, given its demonstrated benefits in neurotic conditions, the most practical option is often to include aspects such as anxiety management within drug counselling sessions from a drug team's community psychiatric nurses.

There are also some general influences on clinical features and progress which are quite characteristic of drug misusers. Often there are high rates of adverse life events, reflecting the direct and indirect complications of a drug-using lifestyle, as well as an effect of personality disorder (Heikkinen et al. 1997, Seivewright et al. 2000b). It must not be assumed that consequences such as adjustment reactions will follow, as drug misusers can appear to take many types of events in their stride, but sometimes the psychiatric effects are significant and this possibility must be anticipated. Impulsive reactions to events are an important factor in self-harm in this population, who have ready access to dangerous methods (Farrell et al. 1996). Personality disorder and depression are both related to self-harm, while general effects of personality disorder are to increase levels of neurotic symptoms (Tyrer et al. 1990) and impair response to psychiatric treatments (Bank & Silk 2001, Mulder 2002). Importantly, studies have shown improvements in psychological disorders such as anxiety and depressive states on methadone maintenance treatment (Musselman & Kell 1995, Calsyn et al. 2000, Teesson et al. 2006). This raises the question (as discussed in Chapter 1) of the mechanism by which methadone produces its benefits, but broadly it would seem that in some cases psychological symptoms are due to drug use and the various associated lifestyle problems. The clinical message is that if moderate depressive or other neurotic features are encountered in the context of starting methadone or buprenorphine treatment, the effects of stabilization should usually be awaited before considering specific psychiatric treatments. Also, marked improvements in psychological state have been demonstrated following detoxification from drugs and other rehabilitation treatments (Craig et al. 1990, Teesson et al. 2006).

Clinicians are sometimes required to make a judgement as to whether drug misuse or a psychiatric disorder is the 'primary' condition, especially where that determines which type of service initially manages an individual. An example might be an amphetamine user whose drug-taking seems linked with problems of depression and lack of confidence. Approaches take into account which condition came first, and careful teasing out of symptoms, but it is also necessary to decide which is currently the major contributor to an individual's various difficulties. In that respect there is a wide spectrum, and certainly those whose drug use is low-level or well-controlled can feel aggrieved when 'all my problems get put down to drugs'. Nevertheless, established drug use tends to exert a powerful influence on an individual's situation and needs, and drug services should, in practical terms, usually operate a low threshold for becoming involved with cases in which it is present to any significant degree. In opiate misusers, non-drug-related counselling or treatment will be unsuccessful if a matter such as consideration for substitute prescribing remains unaddressed.

Personality disorder

In a review of ten years of studies, Verheul et al. (1995) concluded that the best estimate of prevalence of personality disorder in drug misusers was 79%. Most studies were of opiate misusers in treatment, and there is some evidence that the rate is lower across the range of drugs and populations, and outside treatment settings, probably more like 50–60% (Seivewright & Daly 1997, Kokkevi et al. 1998, Grant et al. 2004). The 18% figure found in the ECA study, however, is artificially low, as only a limited range of personality features were rated with the Diagnostic Interview Schedule, which appears to have low validity in drug misusers (Griffin et al. 1987). Some investigators have studied the importance in drug misusers of specific traits seen as part of the spectrum of personality disorder, such as impulsivity and novelty-seeking (Staiger et al. 2007), with these and indeed the differing types of personality disorder seemingly having a degree of biological basis (Widiger et al. 2005).

Making a diagnosis of personality disorder in drug misusers is problematic, due to the particular difficulties of separating true underlying personality disorder from behaviours which develop as part of drug misuse. Most difficulties are with the antisocial behaviours, such as aggressiveness, irresponsibility or tendency to crime, and even in formal diagnostic systems the situation can become rather tautologous. The required approach in both formal and informal rating is to recognize the particular groupings of features which occur in the main categories (those of ASPD or borderline personality disorder are often very apparent in clinical practice), and to take as much account as possible of behaviours which occur independently of drug misuse or cannot be fully explained by it. This includes behaviours prior to dependent drug use, with for instance a history of rebellious behaviour, school absences and petty crime strongly suggesting conduct disorder as a precursor of adult ASPD (Darke et al. 1994b). The term 'secondary' ASPD is sometimes used to describe adult antisocial behaviours which are consequent on drug misuse, but even studies which adopt methods to exclude those features find ASPD to be the most frequent underlying personality disorder. With a colleague I reviewed this subject, examining not only prevalence and the aspect of rating difficulties, but also the effects of personality disorder on outcome and treatment of drug misuse (Seivewright & Daly 1997). Rates of many medical, psychiatric and social complications appear higher in individuals with personality disorder, even including increased rates of HIV infection (Brooner et al. 1993). In most studies causal direction cannot be definitely inferred, but findings such as more injecting, risk behaviours, depression, social impairment and legal problems (Darke et al. 2007) have high face validity, and the direction of findings is very consistent.

When we reviewed the limited evidence regarding treatment, it appeared that personality disorder was associated with worse results in the treatments aimed at abstinence, but had not so marked an effect in methadone maintenance (Gill et al. 1992, Darke et al. 1994b). That pattern of findings, with personality impairment seemingly exerting a less adverse effect in maintenance than various other treatments, has been demonstrated further (van den Bosch & Verheul 2007), even to the point where in populations in which methadone maintenance is the main approach, few overall differences in response are found (Havens & Strathdee 2005, Welch 2007).

As a further phenomenon, several studies have demonstrated improvements in features of personality disorder and associated difficulties in patients on methadone maintenance (Rounsaville et al. 1986, Calsyn et al. 2000, Tremeau et al. 2003), while the borderline personality disorder subjects of Darke et al. (2007), who showed overall higher rates of medical and social problems, did have less tendency to self-harm when in drug treatment. Such effects do seem evident in practice, and no doubt relate to the similar reduction in features such as anxiety and depression noted above. Perhaps the findings of improvements are proof that some of the aspects which are initially included in ratings of personality disorder are features more to do with the complications of drug use itself, but examination of the studies does also strongly suggest a true stabilizing effect of methadone on the more severe personality problems. Once again this would appear to be important clinically, and as buprenorphine becomes more established it will be very interesting to see whether that proves as therapeutic as methadone in relation to personality disorder features. In a conference presentation on this subject I ventured the possibility that some of the improvements may also be 'tactical', whereby addicts in treatment clearly do not show their most aggressive or intimidating features to their prescribing doctors, which if that is considered a manipulation can even be seen as part of the same underlying personality disorder! Indeed other factors are also likely, notably that the reliability of the provision of methadone maintenance leads daily to less stressful situations for the users, who otherwise might tend to 'acting out behaviours' through their low frustration tolerance. Even without formal therapies, some of the general improvements we see in addicts in services are probably due to what can be termed 'behavioural shaping', i.e. the degree of discipline in needing to attend approximately correctly for appointments and other contacts, and be subject there to some containment of antisocial activities.

Much of the treatment of personality disorder is in the psychological sphere, but in an earlier discussion of methadone in this book the poor compliance of drug misusers with formal psychotherapy was noted, and anyway general psychotherapists are reluctant to see those actively involved in substance misuse. Specific psychological approaches that have been demonstrated to be of value in drug misusers with personality disorder include coping skills training (Conrod et al. 2000), dialectical behaviour therapy for those with borderline-type disorder (Linehan et al. 2002), and so-called dual-focus schema therapy (Ball SA 2007), which in effect combines relapse prevention counselling for substance use and cognitive behaviour therapy for personality disorder.

Some forthright but apposite observations were provided a long time ago by an American psychotherapist experienced in counselling individuals with substance abuse and personality disorder, regarding their tendency to use common terms of speech in somewhat loaded and manipulative ways in their dealings with clinicians (Walker 1992a). To me these seem indeed very commonly encountered, even in another country, and it is interesting to speculate whether the usages do strongly suggest personality disorder or whether they are simply in frequent currency among drug misusers in treatment situations generally. Because of the familiarity I have taken the liberty in Table 7.2 of adding my own examples to each of Dr Walker's dictionary and 'SA-PD' meanings of words! A companion paper (Walker 1992b) then looks less at the issues of presentation and more at the therapeutic strategies useful in countering manipulative or self-damaging behaviours. Once again the advice is very prac-tically based and seems pertinent, including the need for clinicians to be truthful with patients and have a reasonably neutral manner in their interactions, to avoid over-identification with the drug-taking scene and slang terms ('these are terms of endearment and should not be modeled by clinicians'), and to set actual limits on the amounts of contact made by demanding individuals in inappropriate circumstances. Reassuringly, the paper even advises the adoption sometimes by clinicians of an air of 'benign stupidity', for instance when wishing to have a patient think through some consequences for themselves, with this apparently known as the 'Columbo approach' after the television detective!

In pharmacological treatment, because of the considerations discussed above there is often the conclusion that substitute prescribing produces the best results in opiate addicts with the added condition of personality disorder, particularly of the antisocial or borderline type. There should also be awareness of treatments which, although not specific for personality disorder, have some demonstrated utility in the condition alongside psychological therapies, including serotonergic antidepressants and low-dose antipsychotics (Markovitz 2004).

Table 7.2 Distortion of common terms by substance abuse–personality disorder (SA-PD) patients

Commonly used word	Common meaning	SA-PD meaning
Help		
As in: 'So you're not going to help me with my sleeping then doctor?'		
	Facilitation, advice, counsel or assistance to a person who must solve a problem	Doing for me what I want in the way I want
Trust		
As in: 'I haven't got proof, I thought you'd trust me after all this time'		
	A feeling of acceptance of another person and a belief that this person will respect one's needs and interests	Accept my version of the truth; believe my story
Rules		
As in: 'That place was hopeless, there were no rules'		
	Basic mechanisms for ensuring order in society	Instructions for other people to follow in dealing with me
Fairness		
As in: 'Well it's not fair if I have to take it in the chemist, I didn't before'		
	Equality and equity in treatment	When things go my way
Work		
As in: 'They're trying to say I should work'		
	Contributing as a means of earning a living	A put-down; a condition of being in an underdog role

Pairs of definitions by Walker (1992a), examples added

Topic in brief – 13. Personality disorder in drug misusers

- Present in about half of addicts, higher rates in treatment populations
- Proper diagnosis requires separation of 'secondary' antisocial behaviours, but antisocial still the highest underlying category
- Adversely affects outcomes in some but not all drug misuse treatments
- Improvements in personality features in individuals on methadone maintenance may be real or artefactual
- Specific pharmacological and psychotherapeutic treatments sometimes useful

Depression

This is another condition which is relatively rarely seen in any 'pure' or simple form, and in drug misusers there is great overlap with low mood caused by social and relationship problems and other adverse circumstances, as well as the ultimately depressive effect of some drugs, or withdrawal states. Furthermore mood can definitely be abnormal through personality disorder alone, and in practice the prescribing of antidepressants to active drug misusers can seem not often fruitful. The users themselves can be disinclined to persist with medications which do not have a quickly beneficial effect, or may even have short-term side-effects, although the sedation from trazodone, mirtazepine, etc., taken at night to aid sleep is typically more valued. If there is reasonably good evidence of the more clinical type of depressive illness there should, however, be adequate trials of medication, to avoid missing a situation which could lead to self-harm or even suicide, common in this group (Oyefeso et al. 1999, Tiet et al. 2006, Ilgen et al. 2007). Indeed in distinguishing actual clinical depression from the low mood from other causes, I have heard it suggested by eminent authorities in this field that suicidal ideation is an important key feature, rather as specific phobic symptoms are in true anxiety disorders (Myrick & Bradey 2001). Reliance should not much be placed on the presence of so-called biological symptoms of depression, as is often done in other psychiatric practice, since poor sleep, feeling better at some times of the day, loss of appetite and weight changes are extremely common in substance misusers for other direct reasons.

Perhaps it is the frequent presence of additional complicating lifestyle factors which makes the literature on depression affecting outcome in drug misuse treatments not as striking as might be expected. A very informative meta-analysis has been provided by Conner et al. (2008), examining studies in which the diagnosis of depression had been made using validated instruments. Overall there was not a significant relationship between depression and future drug use and associated behaviours, although the depressed individuals tended to anyway have the more problematic substance misuse. Among single studies of the various antidepressants one by Carpenter et al. (2004) was particularly interesting, in individuals on methadone still using other drugs with defined depressive disorders. Sertraline was the antidepressant trialled against placebo, with the outcomes, including reduced use of heroin and cocaine, being most significant in those who were not only on the active medication but also had a social environment with less adversity. Another issue which is known to be important from practical general psychiatry is that of 'allegiance effects', i.e. that medications have a better chance of being helpful if the patient is enthusiastic about them at the outset. In our own practice we tend to use the specific serotonergic inhibitors fluoxetine, sertraline or citalopram as first-line, because of both the relative lack of off-putting side-effects compared to the old tricyclics, and also the reported benefits of this group in other 'compulsive' disorders. Exceptions are when we wish to achieve sedation at night, which links in with the desire to preferably avoid benzodiazepines in drug misusers (see Chapter 2).

Drug-induced psychosis

The final area specifically considered here which poses major problems in diagnosis and management is that of drug-induced psychosis, and a helpful editorial in the *British Journal of Psychiatry* was critical of the understanding of this concept (Poole & Brabbins 1996). The authors point out that although '? drug-induced psychosis' is routinely included in the

Table 7.3 Drug-related psychotic reactions

Condition	Possible causative drugs
Intoxication mimicking functional psychosis	Stimulants, cannabis, solvents, ecstasy, LSD
Pathoplastic reactions in functional psychosis	Stimulants, cannabis
Chronic hallucinosis ('flashbacks')	LSD, cannabis
Drug-induced relapse of functional psychosis	Stimulants, cannabis
Withdrawal states	Barbiturates, benzodiazepines

Based on Poole and Brabbins (1996)

differential diagnosis in young psychotic patients, the evidence for lasting psychosis caused by drugs is relatively weak. The monograph on amphetamine psychosis by Connell (1958) is frequently cited, but he apparently confirmed to these authors that he is widely mis-quoted, and that what he demonstrated was that psychotic symptoms precipitated by amphetamines occurred only in relation to intoxication. If the drug is withdrawn, reso-lution of symptoms could be expected, and one of the criticisms is that enduring functional psychoses are not properly diagnosed in drug misusers, as their condition tends to be automatically attributed to drugs. Certainly it is easy to see how, given the high prevalence of drug use in the community, some usage will be genuinely incidental in cases of other psychotic conditions. Table 7.3 indicates the provisional classification of drug-related psychotic reactions suggested in the editorial 'to introduce clarity into a dangerously confused area', all of which fall short of a true enduring disorder.

The listing of drugs potentially causing each condition is based on the availability of some reasonably direct evidence, while the main clinical message is probably that all the drugs listed, with the exception of the sedative–hypnotics mentioned in relation to withdrawal, can cause short-lived psychotic reactions, and also worsen an existing psychotic condition. Importantly, this does not include opiates, while cyclizine and some of the newer stimulants can be added (see Chapter 4). Paranoid ideation following amphetamine or cocaine use is well known, and is typically recognized by users as indicating that they should terminate that episode of usage. The reactions with solvents and LSD are more organic in nature, with visual illusions and hallucinations, and the phenomenon of 'flashbacks' is reasonably well-docu-mented with LSD in particular. With the sedative–hypnotics, psychotic symptoms appear in the withdrawal state rather than as an intoxication effect, although high-dose misuse can definitely cause confusion and disturbed behaviour. In addition to these conditions, pro-longed psychotic reactions may occur when use of the implicated drug itself is ongoing, and such situations can be very troublesome and intractable in clinical practice.

Management has usually been considered to comprise two elements, namely cessation of the drug of misuse and standard antipsychotic drug treatment, as dictated by symptoms. The first can be difficult to achieve, and admission to a psychiatric unit may be necessary to attempt to ensure this (there is still no guarantee), or because of severity of psychosis. Sometimes it is necessary to treat with antipsychotic medication in the face of some known ongoing drug use, in the hope that the medication effect will be over-riding and that, as insight improves, compliance with advice and treatment will generally be better. Medica-tions which act effectively on paranoid symptoms, or which produce sedation, are often particularly indicated. It appears from case reports in the literature that psychotic reactions to ecstasy may sometimes be particularly resistant to treatment (Soar et al. 2004). There is speculation that this may be related to the neurotoxic effects of the drug, but there is no direct evidence and, in practice, the same treatment approaches have to be used.

Although criticism of the concept of drug-induced psychosis is clearly justified, it remains possible that a psychosis could be substantially caused by drugs and persist in the absence of drug use. Claims have been made in this regard for cannabis, initially by Andreasson et al. (1987), with several large-scale and long-term studies showing increased rates of what appears to be true schizophrenia in individuals with heavy cannabis use histories (Arseneault et al. 2004, Arendt et al. 2005, Moore et al. 2007). It is usually considered likely that some kind of vulnerability is at work in those who do develop schizophrenia or a closely related condition with exposure to cannabis (Verdoux 2004), while in terms of the product used there are considerations of strength (Smith 2005) and ratio of different cannabinoid constituents (Morgan & Curran 2008). In practice there do seem cases in whom a psychotic reaction persists for weeks, or even months, after all evidence suggests drug use has stopped, and the question arises as to how long such a period needs to be before symptoms should be deemed to indicate a functional psychosis, an area considered by Flaum and Schultz (1996). With amphetamine, in contrast to the original findings by Connell referred to above, it seems that some substance-induced psychoses can indeed persist in the absence of ongoing use, through brain mechanisms best described as forms of sensitivity to drug exposure (Curran et al. 2004). It may also be that drugs can lead to fuller expression of psychotic features in a case of latent or developing psychosis, or in an individual who is constitutionally susceptible by virtue of family history, previous abnormal experiences or schizoid personality (Henquet et al. 2005), but such relationships are difficult to demonstrate, and the systematic evidence is still building. In a relatively early review Boutros and Bowers (1996) concluded that across a range of drugs a threshold-lowering effect does occur, and it may well be that the vulnerability factors particularly being tested at the present time in relation to cannabis are more widely applicable.

Topic in brief – 14. Drug-induced psychosis

- Different drugs produce different psychotic syndromes, with no psychosis directly from opiates
- Most reactions are short-lived if drugs withdrawn, but various mechanisms can prolong symptoms
- Much persuasion often required for paranoid individuals to take medication
- With generally high prevalence of drug misuse, some detected use is incidental in individuals developing 'core' psychotic illnesses

Drug misuse in the severely mentally ill

Particular reasons to account for drug misuse by people with schizophrenia, manic depressive psychosis and other severe mental illnesses may be classed as broadly social, or individual. As institutionalization decreases there is greater exposure to available drugs in the community; some community placements in cities, and other accommodation which the severely mentally ill may be offered, are in areas of high drug prevalence. Also, people with an obvious vulnerability can be exploited by drug dealers, who may for instance give drugs free initially in order to gain a regular customer over whom they have easy control.

At an individual level, a person with severe mental illness is likely to have impairments in the processes of judgement and insight which usually afford some control against drug-taking. They may then find that drugs actually alleviate some of their symptoms, with cannabis or heroin perhaps providing some relief from hallucinations or troublesome side-effects of medication, or stimulants giving energy in a person with negative symptoms. Clinicians would see this as outweighed by the propensity of drugs to directly worsen psychosis, and the adverse influence on psychiatric treatments, but it can be very difficult to discourage drug use when a patient perceives short-term benefits. It may be possible for some individuals to reproduce symptoms which are pleasurable, or they may value the degree of control over their symptoms which drug use brings. Being part of the drugs scene can provide a social role and opportunities for interaction with people which are otherwise lacking, and it is necessary to counter this by involvement in non-drug-related activities as part of treatment.

As well as these general effects, features which distinguish those among the severely mentally ill who are likely to misuse drugs have been investigated. Mueser et al. (1997) found antisocial personality disorder to be a risk factor, just as it is for developing drug misuse generally (see above). Males are more prone, again reflecting the general pattern in drug misuse, and where females do have dual diagnosis they have been found to have more social contact and fewer legal problems, but more violent victimization and medical illness than men (Brunette & Drake 1997).

In the large Epidemiologic Catchment Area study in the community referred to above (Regier et al. 1990) 28% of those with schizophrenia were found to have drug dependence or abuse, but at that time Galanter et al. (1994) pointed out that such studies do not reflect the major burden that dual diagnosis patients place upon clinical services. From their perspective in New York they suggested that 'the considerable impact of these patients is better reflected in the prevalence of substance abuse in emergency rooms, psychiatric units, medical services and perinatal programs', with 34% of all general hospital psychiatric admissions in New York State assessed as being dually diagnosed (Haugland et al. 1991). In studies since then, in London, Menezes et al. (1996) assessed all patients with psychotic illness who had had contact with the mental health services in a geographical sector, and found a one-year prevalence rate for any substance problem of 36%. Young male subjects had the highest rates, at 50% in the 20–29 age group for drug misuse alone. Rates of this order for substance misuse among individuals with psychosis have since been repeatedly demonstrated (Graham et al. 2001, Kavanagh et al. 2002, Weaver et al. 2003), and a review article specifically on cannabis use prevalence by Green et al. (2005) carefully analyses the reasons for the range of rates, such as sampling.

As would be expected, the additional aspect of drug misuse has been shown to complicate the progress of those with severe mental illness, in and outside treatment. Thus, the dually diagnosed have been found to have increased levels of violence (Cuffell et al. 1994, Scott et al. 1998, Soyka 2000), hostile behaviour (Bartels et al. 1991), offending (Lehman et al. 1993, Scott et al. 1998), family problems (Lehman et al. 1993), homelessness, various poor prognosis features (Swofford et al. 1996, Hunt et al. 2002, Margolese et al. 2004) and illness and injury (Dickey et al. 2000), in comparison with individuals with psychosis only. There often appears to be poorer compliance with treatments including antipsychotic medication, although a reported pattern of increased use of inpatient services after deterioration and higher overall treatment costs is in some doubt (Menezes et al. 1996, Tyrer & Weaver 2004). Another indication that the profile of

Table 7.4 Principles of treatment of drug misuse in the severely mentally ill

Assertive outreach
Visit at home or other places as necessary. Stress benefits of contact and treatment to patient and significant others
Close monitoring
Particularly necessary in difficult cases. Opportunities to do this may be presented by sheltered housing, day hospitals, probation, etc.
Integration
Linking between general psychiatric and substance misuse services
Comprehensiveness
Address practical issues, e.g. activities, benefits, social skills, as well as clinical disorders
Stable living situation
Direct efforts towards this, otherwise progress is unlikely
Flexibility
Modify the traditional approach to addiction counselling
Stage-wise treatment
Recognize which stage of treatment is applicable – engagement/persuasion/active treatment/relapse prevention
Longitudinal perspective
Recognize that drug misuse is a chronic relapsing disorder
Optimism
Counter demoralization among patients, families and treatment providers

Based on Drake et al. (1993, 2001)

problems is not all one-way, i.e. worse in dual diagnosis cases, was a study finding that although the latter showed the more overt behavioural disturbances, they had better preservation of social competence than other psychotic patients, perhaps in effect less deterioration with 'negative' symptoms (Penk et al. 2000). While many of the associated problems may partly reflect lifestyle aspects of drug misuse, or in some cases underlying personality features, the increasing evidence for use of drugs directly worsening psychosis has been examined at various stages in this book.

Principles of treatment

A group of clinical researchers in New Hampshire, USA, who are highly experienced in the treatment of substance abuse in the severely mentally ill have identified certain key principles of management (Drake et al. 1993, 2001), which are shown in Table 7.4. They consider that a special approach is necessary because the severely mentally ill do not identify problems in the same way, they typically have difficulty with addiction treatment approaches such as group therapy, and there is an ever-present danger that this group fall between two sets of services. Their work is in a unit specifically for dual diagnosis patients, and although as will be seen much treatment is now more community-based, the principles ring true as being generally applicable in working with this patient group.

Many will recognize the appropriateness of these suggested measures, especially being flexible in terms of opportunities for contact, helping with practical aspects and activities as far as possible, and adapting routine treatment situations. It is also beneficial to form good links with family, partner or anyone else who provides important support to the patient, as they may help in areas such as detecting drug use, managing medication, or compliance with appointments. As with the patient, a broad approach which addresses practical difficulties as well as the clinical conditions is often valued.

Some of the problems of acceptability and compliance in drug misuse treatment may be less in those countries outside the USA where treatment is more pragmatic, and not so uniformly based on the 12-step approach and group therapy, which the severely mentally ill can find off-putting. However, any counselling can be difficult in those with impaired cognitive abilities, and it is unfortunate that there are so few useful pharmacological treatments for non-opiate misuse, which is frequently encountered in this population. If the drug misuse is of opiates, it is tempting to use methadone because this often facilitates engagement and provides a degree of symptomatic stability, but probably the criteria for maintenance on methadone or other opioids should be similar to those for anybody else.

The only really controversial one of these principles is integration, as these clinical researchers favour a team specifically and solely treating dual diagnosis cases, providing the general psychiatric and substance misuse input. This model will next be described, while in current community treatment in many countries the 'intregation' would be actually liaison, between workers and units for the two specialities. The policies which lie behind dual diagnosis service provision in the UK are included in an authoritative review by Abou-Saleh (2007), and again some main examples of community treatments follow here.

Ultra-specialist treatment units

The same New Hampshire group have described 'continuous treatment teams' (Drake et al. 1996), who treat the dual diagnosis patients, with 24-hour responsibility for case management. There is a flexible approach to individual and group therapy, the latter being either educational or treatment-oriented in the case of those committed to abstinence. There is a practical focus on social situation, social skills and aspects of daily living.

Behaviour therapy techniques have also been used with such dual diagnosis patients, to address symptom management, medication management, recreation and leisure, and social skills (Jerrell & Ridgeley 1995). In New York City there has been a combined service comprising a locked ward, a halfway house and a day programme, the operation and results of which were described by Galanter et al. (1994). This work was with a particularly challenging population, mostly disadvantaged minorities, homeless, and using crack cocaine. The inpatient unit included a token economy system to encourage compliance and participation in therapy, while other elements of the service were a peer leadership approach, educational groups, 12-step addiction groups, and conventional antipsychotic treatment.

Jerrell and Ridgeley (1995) compared three approaches – case management, behaviour therapy, and the 12-step model – at a follow-up of two years, and there was a suggestion, within generally encouraging results over 18 months, that behaviour therapy had the most effect, and 12-step treatment the least. In a number of studies expertly provided ultra-specialist treatment along the lines described has been found to be superior to various kinds of standard treatments (Drake et al. 2001, 2007), but clearly not many areas have dual diagnosis services in full form. It might be thought that there is now enough evidence to at least promote some major elements of the dual diagnosis treatment discussed above, although purists can point to a systematic review which concluded that it was not possible to demonstrate a definite advantage for any set model of treatment provision (Ley et al. 2001).

Johnson (1997) critically examined whether ultra-specialist services should be adopted outside the USA, in particular in Europe. She pointed out that such a specialized service covering a large geographical area could cut across some of the strong links formed between psychiatric services and primary care in smaller localities, which is a basic approach in community psychiatry in the UK and other countries. There is also the common dilemma that the more specialized the unit, the more it may discourage others from attempting treatment at all for that patient group. She concluded that it may be preferable to investigate ways of delivering care for dual diagnosis patients within established community mental health teams rather than to form distinct specialist teams. The theme of marked differences transatlantically in the prevailing ethos of services has been examined further (Fiander et al. 2003), and many dual diagnosis projects have been established in ways other than full integrated provision.

Other treatment models

It could be argued that if there are existing teams in an area for substance misuse and general psychiatry, with a good number of community-based workers plus available inpatient facilites, there should be no need for any special initiatives to manage individuals who have two conditions. Common sense might dictate that if a person with a psychotic condition and drug misuse was experiencing more problems with severe delusional phenomena and other signs of illness, then the concentration of input at that time would be from general psychiatry, whereas if initiation of drug treatment was required or there were particular developments with that or additional substance usage, drug workers would be to the fore. To a large extent this probably happens in practice, but virtually wherever the subject of dual diagnosis is discussed the issue of 'falling through the gap' between the two types of services is identified (e.g. el-Guebaly 2004). Most clinicians will be familiar with this potential problem, while in drug misuse we perhaps bear the burden of covering both aspects relatively often, for instance when somebody with schizophrenia who is on methadone keeps engaged with the drug service, but drops out of their appointments for general psychiatric care. If we operate psychiatric drug misuse services we ought to be able to handle that situation to some extent, for instance managing the antipsychotic prescribing, but on the other hand there will be times when acute emergencies occur and when the question arises of admission to a general unit, perhaps compulsorily. There does therefore need to be a commitment on the part of both general psychiatric and substance misuse services to continue involvement whatever the severity of the respective conditions, as long as both kinds of treatments remain indicated. This is much more in the area of liaison rather than actual integration of services, and at local level policies need to be drawn up to ensure that satisfactory and usually joint management occurs. This is the area which from a UK perspective in particular has been examined by Abou-Saleh (2007), while the need for additional training of both types of workers who encounter dual diagnosis patients is also frequently pointed out (Maslin et al. 2001, Drake et al. 2007).

It is increasingly common to have specific dual diagnosis worker posts within teams, based in either of the types of service. Those authorities who consider that the problematic impact of dual diagnosis is most strongly seen in acute and emergency general psychiatry, or indeed in casualty departments, would tend to favour the attachment to psychiatric rather than drug services, especially since psychotic patients are known to be under-represented in routine drug caseloads. One such development was set up and carefully evaluated by Griffin et al. (2008), and these clinicians were of the opinion regarding the two dual diagnosis community psychiatric nurse posts that 'their full integration within the community mental health teams was crucial in providing the necessary level of staff trust and support'.

There is no doubt that even within community provision the principles of management identified by the ultra-specialist researchers as described above are frequently drawn upon, and a further literature is developing on specific interventions that can be included in treatment. These include tailored forms of cognitive therapy (Graham 1998) and motivational interviewing (Martino et al. 2006), and various types of family intervention (Kavanagh et al. 2000, Haddock et al. 2003). In general it can be stated that the most standard pharmacological treatments for substance dependence, therefore mainly on opiates and alcohol, remain indicated in dual diagnosis patients, as do the medications for severe mental illness. Within the former, there often seems a suspicion in practice that methadone will be particularly stabilizing in opiate-dependent individuals with psychotic illness, but there is no real evidence to suggest that buprenorphine will not be as beneficial if its standard benefits occur. Regarding antipsychotics, some studies suggest particular effectiveness of clozapine in the dually diagnosed, but on the other hand clinicians can be concerned about using this rather than more routine antipsychotic medications because a greater degree of monitoring for blood abnormalities and side-effects is necessary. Available evidence regarding this and other medications for substance misuse and psychiatric disorder in dual diagnosis has been further reviewed by Crome and Myton (2007).

Topic in brief – 15. Managing drug misuse in the severely mentally ill

- Much flexibility required in all aspects, from engagement onwards
- Often important to counter patients' beliefs that substance use simply relieves their illness
- Principles identified from ultra-specialist units are useful, but most treatment now more community-based
- Where indicated, the use of pharmacological drug misuse treatments is less affected by illness than counselling approaches

8 Providing clinical services
Liaison work and special patient groups

Introduction

The aim of this final chapter is to highlight some aspects of treatment of conditions that are frequently associated with drug misuse, and more especially the features of actual management of drug problems in individuals with those conditions, or in particular settings. The predominant associated conditions which are highly relevant for community drug services are the associated psychiatric disorders, especially when the drug service is a psychiatrically based one, and these have already been discussed. Drug misusers also frequently find themselves on medical wards with various physical complications, while the very serious infectious complications of HIV and hepatitis have required much liaison work and indeed major changes in drug policy. The threat of HIV being substantially transmitted via injecting drug misusers from the original risk groups to the general heterosexual community meant that drug misuse treatment took on a more public health orientation, and then more recently there has been a second 'wave' of developments linked with another agenda for treatment services, that of crime reduction. In the UK at least, treatment in prisons used to be very separate from community treatment as practised by National Health Service clinicians, but this is an area where once again there have been developments in terms of liaison. Also many drug services have special projects for young users and clinics for pregnant addicts, and some of the issues which appear important in practice in relation to such patient populations will be briefly reviewed.

The general hospital

Unless there is excellent liaison, many problems can occur when drug misusers not in current treatment are admitted to general hospital wards for a physical disorder. Quite often of course the presenting condition is a direct complication of drug misuse, such as deep vein thrombosis, pulmonary embolus, endocarditis or severe ulceration, but even when a person's addiction has been severe enough to produce these they will not necessarily be in contact with a drug service. Sometimes the first that is known of the individual is a call from a medical ward, perhaps to say that some behaviour problems or dispute have emerged with no substitute medication prescribed, and the addict becoming agitated with withdrawal symptoms. It can be difficult for ward doctors to know what to prescribe, even if the initial stage of confirmation of opiate dependence with instant urine testing has been satisfactorily completed. Thinking of the opiate addicts in particular, who are indeed overall the most likely group to develop the conditions indicated above, the doctors on a medical unit can be wary of methadone, because of its particular implications and administrative complications, while starting buprenorphine is also somewhat difficult, and hospital wards are one of the settings where sometimes dihydrocodeine can be useful for a period.

At other times there may be no notification of an addict being on the general ward until it is time for discharge, and then the drug service is faced with taking somebody on immediately for prescribing with little time for assessment, and one or other medication option already established. Certainly over the years that I have been practising our services have often received a telephone call saying that somebody we do not know is going to be discharged from their medical treatment, with methadone prescribed on the ward, and requesting that we take them on for continuation.

Mention is made of these issues really to emphasize the need for more than just telephone liaison, but a model of 'inreach' of drug workers to the medical, surgical and other wards. Some services are just able to provide a worker to go to the ward when called, but in one of our areas we have two nurse specialists in drug misuse actually based in the general hospital, to receive notification on any day of individuals who have been admitted who will require drug misuse assessment and treatment. Sometimes the patients are known to us, and it will be easier for these workers attached to the hospital to obtain details of current medication from the drug team – or the local pharmacy where they attend is always the most direct source, including of information on whether the medication for the day of admission was collected. Other inpatients will not be known to our service, and we find it preferable to have our workers 'on the spot' to do an assessment and advise on the ward, rather than simply relying on telephone calls or an urgent need for assessment at the drug team base when a patient has just been discharged. We have even established the process whereby the doctors from medicine, surgery, etc. will issue the community prescriptions for daily dispensing of methadone or buprenorphine at a local pharmacy, which in theory any doctor can do but is actually very rarely done by nonspecialists unless such tuition is provided. This enables any gap between discharge (for instance at a weekend) and drug team appointment to be bridged without interruption of substitute medication, although in the particular area where we have this development such waits are anyway brief.

Treatment in pregnancy

This is another field in which there are often workers allocated from a drug service to have a role with the particular patient group. Many drug services will have special clinics for the pregnant users, perhaps including the period after childbirth for a few months, because of the ongoing similar issues which will still be relevant (Day et al. 2003). Increasingly services in the UK have individuals dually trained in midwifery and in substance misuse, perhaps with a general nursing qualification as well, to play a leading part in the setting up of the special provision, with social workers experienced in work with children, including child protection. Often one of the obstetricians in the local district will also specialize to some extent in managing the pregnant drug misusers, with further direct opportunities for liaison and joint sessions.

A short review of substance misuse during pregnancy, including adverse effects in pregnancy and by association in children later, and screening and management, has been published by Johnson et al. (2003). Some of the aspects most relevant for drug services are indicated in Table 8.1. There is concentration here on opiate-dependent women, as clinical treatments have the most application in that group, but drug services must be able to advise users on other drugs also, with cocaine for instance producing exceptionally high rates of obstetric complications (Fajemirokun-Odudeyi & Lindow 2004), and links found between cannabis use in early pregnancy and childhood cancer (Bluhm et al. 2006). I have mentioned that social workers are attached to drug services in the clinics for pregnant women,

Table 8.1 Treatment of pregnant opiate misusers

Presentation
Often late
May be sensitive about statutory involvement
Associated features
Other risk factors for adverse fetal development
Partner often using drugs
Liaison
Antenatal and medical services
Social services
Treatment
Methadone where indicated, maintenance suitable but sometimes detoxification if requested
Buprenorphine safe and associated with less neonatal withdrawal
Avoid benzodiazepines

which relates to the primacy of child protection in UK policies and legislation, and so clearly something of a balancing act needs to be struck to avoid possible evasion of presentation by addicts fearful of official action.

Quick detoxifications should not be undertaken in pregnancy, since significant opiate withdrawal stimulates uterine motility, with risk therefore of miscarriage in the early stages or premature labour in the later. It has typically been advised that where detoxification is attempted the process should be in the middle trimester where the risk from uterine stimulation is somewhat less, but anyway any reduction should not be at all sudden. Because of the benefits of good fetal weight, fewer complications and increased general stability, maintenance on the same dose of methadone or buprenorphine is increasingly recommended, but this does present a genuine dilemma in women who definitely want to be off substitute medication at delivery time. The emergence of buprenorphine as a direct alternative to methadone in all opioid substitution treatment, as discussed in detail elsewhere in the book, may have a strong influence on treatment in pregnancy, as there is now much evidence regarding its safety, and it does seem that neonatal withdrawal symptoms when the mother is still on medication at the birth are less with buprenorphine than with methadone (Fischer et al. 2000, Lacroix et al. 2004).

An excellent fuller review of all the main aspects of managing drug misuse in pregnancy has been provided by Day and George (2007).

Young drug users

Once again many areas have special services for this group, not necessarily clinical in nature. Much substance abuse in adolescents is of alcohol, cannabis, ecstasy, LSD, etc., with (as reviewed in Chapter 4) far fewer clinical treatment implications than there are in opiate dependence. Helping services may be from nonstatutory agencies, including youth workers, with much attention to lifestyle factors, counselling regarding personal or family problems, and enabling non-drug activities. Some counselling interventions are systematic in nature, with one trial of cognitive-behavioural coping skills and psychoeducation therapies finding reasonable effectiveness, with less good outcomes in adolescents with additional conduct disorder (Kaminer et al. 2002).

Conduct disorder is indeed one of the conditions most strongly associated with adolescent substance misuse, and is related to broadly the same range of background factors in its origins. These have been discussed in the introductory chapter of this book and also the section on personality disorder, which condition often continues from the behaviours shown in adolescent conduct disorder. Quite often parental substance misuse is present, typically of alcohol where the young person has turned instead to drugs, and a careful examination of the genetic, social and behavioural elements in such links has been provided by Gilvarry and Crome (2004).

In some ways management of heroin dependence in adolescents is less problematic than in adults, because by definition histories are usually shorter and the actual condition less severe. However, on the other hand, for young people to be using heroin there may often be very significant distress from associated problems such as those within the family, with traumatic early events perhaps having occurred. Also there is very unlikely to be any fully formed motivation in an adolescent that they definitely want to be free of substance use, or even the problematic heroin use, and it is questionable whether the forms of motivational interviewing used in adults are very appropriate. In a study which initially included 200 young people in London there were promising early effects after one type of motivational interviewing, especially on cannabis use, but when most of the individuals were followed up a year later the differences between the intervention group and controls had almost entirely disappeared (McCambridge & Strang 2005).

In a detoxification lofexidine is frequently used in the UK, and buprenorphine seems to have inherently more appeal than methadone if longer-term treatment is required. There has always been some reluctance to use methadone in the young, because of its sheer potency and the tendency for treatment to become lengthy even when that was not the original intention, with then much discomfort in withdrawal attempts. Many adolescents might not 'qualify' for methadone in programmes due to relatively brief duration of opiate dependence, although of course some adolescents have had full dependence on heroin for four or five years, and methadone is sometimes necessary where buprenorphine seems unsuitable for any reason. Certainly drug services must accept that long-term opioid prescribing may quite often be required, with younger patients showing particularly high relapse rates in some studies (Kaminer 2002). Within this age range there will be good and poor prognosis cases, and some of the patterns of progress which we find in our own services in detoxification work have been discussed in Chapter 3. As indicated there, lofexidine is used rather than clonidine, while the latter compared unfavourably to buprenorphine in a randomized trial in young people (Marsch et al. 2005).

Topic in brief – 16. Drug misuse in adolescents

- Only requires specific clinical treatments in a minority of cases
- Much other management can be from a range of services, with emphasis on forms of counselling and enabling non-drug activities
- Is strongly associated with conduct disorders, which can both require treatment and affect drug treatment outcomes
- May lead to established heroin dependence, with buprenorphine often a suitable approach

Older users

It is also being recognized that there are problems at the other end of the age range, even within routinely deployed drug services. The concern here is not the well-recognized one of alcohol and benzodiazepine dependence in the elderly, which lies outside the scope of this book, but the issue of more of our general caseload being on substitution treatment well into middle age (which is not itself problematic) and having demonstrably high rates of additional psychological and particularly physical health difficulties (Gossop & Moos 2008). With study evidence emerging on this issue, there is concern that in modern-day drug clinics geared towards 'mass' treatment and immediate referral schemes such as those for released prisoners (see below), there may be insufficient time to attend to the complications which develop. Good management of additional physical disorders is considered one of the potential benefits of primary care treatment for drug dependence, but as has been noted there are often difficulties even in managing the presenting drug misuse in those appointments, and primary care specialist services usually have the same approach of seeing the maximum number of users on a harm-reduction basis as do the other specialist clinics. So far drug services have not provided special arrangements for patients with simply more physical problems in the way that they have done for other user groups, but this is perhaps increasingly necessary. At a very practical level workers often have to make exceptions in controlled drug dispensing arrangements for those with mobility problems, with most policy recommendations clearly having younger fully mobile users in mind.

Pain management

Something of a stereotype now follows, but in a good cause: to illustrate some practical points in management of minor opioid misuse. I would contend that there is a syndrome of a classic case of someone who becomes dependent on paracetamol and codeine combinations, or dihydrocodeine, dextropropoxyphene or something similar, with the following features:

- Young middle-aged to middle-aged women
- Some psychological or relationship problems
- Opioid initially started for a painful condition
- Sometimes benzodiazepine or alcohol misuse, and often antidepressant prescribing
- No inclination to use of 'street' drugs

Perhaps sub-cultural and gender aspects are important in this form of drug misuse, with the tranquillizing and slight euphoriant effects of minor opioids being valued in those who would be disinclined to go drinking with friends, or still less take illicit drugs. Often the minor opioids have been started by a primary care physician because of back pain, abdominal problems or tension headaches, and then escalation of usage can occur, with presentation early for supplies and the doctor realising that consumption is unduly high. Of course males and older (or younger) people can be affected, but the profile above does have some backing from studies (e.g. Hughes et al. 1999).

Efforts are put into preventing minor opioid misuse, both in primary care policies and in pharmacy schemes to reduce inappropriate sale of 'over-the-counter' products (McBride et al. 2003). In treatment, this is an example of a population usually disinclined to take methadone, which resonates with the USA literature recommending buprenorphine for the 'new' 'middle-class' addicts who would not go to methadone clinics (Mitka 2003). In our services we find the supportive aspects of drug counselling important in this group, along with systematic advice from the same workers on reducing consumption, and liaison with prescribers. With such elements in place some individuals can simply comply with a reducing course of their index drug, but often a switch to buprenorphine is useful as it is new to the user and therefore avoids established anxieties about going below a certain dose of their medication.

A different problematic situation is when individuals with established opiate dependence then develop a painful condition, which indeed they do more than most people partly because of complications of drug abuse. Even a condition such as severe leg ulceration can lead to requests for analgesics strong enough to work in an individual who is already on opioid maintenance treatment, with high tolerance. The analgesic effect of methadone, potent though it is, is typically discounted in such requests, although there may separately be enthusiasm for covering both issues with an increase in methadone from others involved with the patient, who wish to avoid giving anything additional.

This situation is almost always difficult to manage, and ultimately there is no getting around the fact that one of the things that is compromised when an individual uses and becomes dependent on heroin is the straightforward relief of pain for which opioids would normally be used. Guidelines tend to recommend the use of non-opioid methods of pain relief, including non-steroidal analgesics, low-dose antidepressants, transcutaneous electrical nerve stimulation, acupuncture or physiotherapy, following full assessment to establish any underlying cause of the pain. Sometimes splitting of methadone dose is useful, with the analgesic effect thought to be increased if this is done rather than taking the day's dose in one.

In a review of the management of pain in patients receiving maintenance methadone or buprenorphine Alford et al. (2006) point out the fear that some non-drug clinicians may have that if they give an opioid, this could cause the patient to relapse into drug abuse. The reviewers suggest that it is actually the converse situation, i.e. inadequate relief of pain and ongoing symptoms, that is more associated with relapse, and they also indicate that the risks of combining more than one opioid are not great specifically when pain is present. Sometimes drug teams are referred patients who have, however, been prescribed extremely large doses of morphine in a pain clinic, where relying on patients' own subjective description of their symptoms is implicit in assessment. In such circumstances the point applies which has been made in the chapter on alternative medications to methadone, that conversions to an opioid substitute for stabilization or withdrawal can be done at more conservative doses of our treatments than comparison tables would suggest.

HIV and hepatitis

It was the threat of widespread transmission of HIV that led to national policy recommendations for more maintenance opioid substitution treatment to be used in the UK, as part of a package of 'harm-reduction' measures. Two decades on there appears little doubt that the overall approach in this country was successful in limiting HIV rates in injecting addicts (Farrell et al. 2005), although with voluntary testing the true prevalence is unknown, and may possibly be rising at the present time. The resources provided at the time of the major public health concerns have meant that much practical support is available to positive patients, even to the point of special housing, and psychological support is provided by staff attached to genito-urinary medicine departments.

The presence of HIV does not fundamentally affect the direct treatments for drug misuse, but with increasing illness there may be similar issues to those in the older addicts with other physical diseases, which have been discussed. When HIV antiviral therapy is given there may be some reduced efficacy of methadone through increased metabolism (Akerele et al. 2002), but if this seems to be so the dose can readily be increased. As more injecting drug users who became infected despite the preventive measures actually become ill with the disease, it is necessary for workers to have some knowledge of the treatments which are applied.

The impression of better survival than was at first feared is correct, with the prognosis of HIV having greatly improved due to the routine use of triple antiretroviral therapy. Many of the medications now used can be given just once a day, and side-effects are much less than with the early treatments (Gazzard et al. 2005). The decision of when to start treatment has usually been based on specific values in the blood counts, and as the medications have become easier to tolerate it has not necessarily been to patients' disadvantage if treatment in the days of the earlier drug options was delayed (Phillips et al. 2007).

A much more common problem in caseloads of drug services is hepatitis C, which appears to be more transmissible than HIV and therefore not as well prevented by the harm-reduction initiatives such as needle and syringe provision schemes. This is also treated by antiretroviral drugs, and there has gradually been increased inclusion of injecting drug users in treatment programmes (Schaefer et al. 2004). Testing is routinely carried out within drug services, and if patients prove positive there is one aspect of progress which we must assess especially carefully, i.e. alcohol consumption. There is no doubt that heavy drinking does much worsen the prognosis of hepatitis C, rendering progression to the cirrhosis stage of the disease far more likely (Pessione et al. 1998), and the situations which are associated with heavy drinking in drug misusers must be guarded against. As indicated in the section on alcohol in Chapter 4 these often include the periods of adjustment to being without euphoriant drugs in a monitored treatment programme, and prescribing regimes need to be in sufficient dosage (and sometimes combination) to give individuals the best chance of avoiding all substances, including alcohol. The diagnosis of hepatitis C being known to a patient can have an impact on their alcohol consumption (McCusker 2001), and the importance regarding prognosis should certainly be made very clear. A thorough review of treatment aspects of hepatitis C infection in methadone maintenance patients has been provided by Novick and Creek (2008).

Topic in brief – 17. Hepatitis C

- Has proved much more transmissible than HIV, especially by sharing injecting equipment
- Prevalence rates in populations of injectors are often over 50%, and testing should be available in all clinical drug services
- Can remain a mild disease but alcohol misuse much worsens the prognosis
- Treatment is increasingly available, with relatively well-tolerated medications

Treatment in prisons

Being in prison is undoubtedly very different to living in the outside world, and it is not surprising that different approaches to managing drug problems have been in place. There has been much debate as to whether injecting equipment and even condoms should be made available in prisons because of disease transmission risks, but in some ways it is much more difficult to do that than in the general population. There is often not a great deal of general sympathy for addicts in custody, as the setting is partly geared towards punishment for crimes, and if an offender has also been using illegal drugs and so goes into withdrawal, many might think that to be their just desserts. Certainly there has been little enthusiasm for implementing all aspects of community drug services for addict prisoners, and opioid maintenance treatment has been quite rare in the UK until recently. The addict is, after all, in a restricted setting, and arguably should take the opportunity to become clean of drugs – in fact some users will say this is exactly what they want to do.

It is known, however, that drugs are readily available in many prisons, and the rate of adverse incidents and the time and effort spent in detecting smuggling of drugs in has been enough to persuade some authorities that at least the basics of treatment should be available. The most routine option has become to provide a detoxification for opiate misusers, with for instance lofexidine or dihydrocodeine, and also benzodiazepines will often be issued if there is a history of abuse of these and it is intended to avoid the possibility of fits with a short withdrawal course. The adverse incidents in custody and prisons have included some deaths in users of crack cocaine, with physical explanations postulated but no very satisfactory treatment for cocaine withdrawal indicated. Prison services have typically been wary of methadone, and in favouring lofexidine use it was encouraging that a randomized double-blind trial carried out by prison specialists found lofexidine to be as effective as methadone in relief of withdrawal symptoms (Howells et al. 2002).

Gradually, however, there have been increased calls for opioid maintenance to be made available to prisoners, partly as the hepatitis C figures highlighted the risks of becoming infected when no treatment is available. Even syringe exchange programmes have been introduced in some countries, and a review of studies of these found reports of drug use to remain stable or decrease, no new cases of HIV, hepatitis B or C transmission, and 'no reports of serious unintended negative events, such as initiation of injection or the use of needles as weapons' (Dolan et al. 2003). Regarding opioid maintenance, a major stimulus to the introduction of this was a series of demonstrations of hugely increased death rates in heroin addicts very shortly after release from prison (Bird & Hutchinson 2003, Farrell & Marsden 2008). A classic situation, which is well known but was re-appraised in the light of these demonstrations, is of a heroin addict who comes off their drug in prison, with opiate tolerance therefore going down, but is then tempted to take their previously usual amount when back at liberty, with fatal results. It was considered that if a highly tolerant opiate addict went to prison it was simply too dangerous to detoxify them unrealistically, with substitution treatment therefore provided in many areas. Methadone, buprenorphine or sometimes other opioids can be given, and, as well as the standard benefits of substitution treatment ensuing, follow-up of individuals provided with methadone maintenance has shown ongoing reductions in mortality, re-incarceration and hepatitis C infection (Dolan et al. 2005).

One of the studies of the greatly increased death rate of recently released addict prisoners (Farrell & Marsden 2008) had as a conclusion that there must be 'planned referral to community-based treatment services'. Coming full circle, in our main service we offer first-day appointments for released prisoners from our area to continue their substitution treatment, or naltrexone in cases where that has already been selected by a user and started.

APPENDIX: PROTOCOLS FOR QUICK DETOXIFICATION FROM HEROIN

These protocols relate to treatment as described on pages 62–64. This is the form in which information is given to patients, except for the additional notes.

Method 1 – Symptomatic medication

These medications are to be taken only if required

Diazepam (5 mg tablets) (reduces muscle cramps, anxiety and cravings)

Take tablets one or two at a time, with at least 4 hours between doses.
  Maximum daily dose:

Day	No. of tablets
1	2
2	4
3	6
4	6
5	4
6	2
7	1
Total	25 tablets

Zopiclone (7.5 mg tablets) (helps sleep)

Unfortunately sleep may be poor even with these sleeping tablets. Do not take more than the recommended dose, as this can be dangerous and is unlikely to be effective.
  Maximum dose – two tablets at night. Total 14 tablets.

Buscopan (10 mg tablets) (reduces stomach spasm)

Take tablets two at a time, with at least 4 hours between doses.
  Maximum dose – eight tablets in 24 hours. Total 30 tablets.

Lomotil (2.5 mg tablets) (reduces diarrhoea)

Ensure plenty of fluids are taken during any periods of diarrhoea and/or vomiting.

Take four tablets initially, when diarrhoea starts, then two tablets every 6 hours until it stops. Total 30 tablets.

Note: To avoid over-use of medication and to facilitate contact, the total medication supply may be divided into two prescriptions, with the worker providing the second one 2 to 3 days into the detoxification.

Method 2 – Lofexidine plus symptomatic medication

All medications are to be taken only if required

Lofexidine (0.2 mg tablets) (treatment for withdrawal symptoms)

Take tablets at regular intervals, as shown. The following are the *maximum* doses. Remember to check your pulse before each dose and take the medication only if it is above 60 beats/minute.

	9:00 am	1:00 pm	5:00 pm	9:00 pm	Total tablets in 24 hours
Day 1	2	2	2	2	8
Day 2	3	2	2	3	10
Day 3	3	3	3	3	12
Day 4	3	3	3	3	12
Day 5	3	2	2	3	10
Day 6	2	2	2	2	8
Day 7	—	—	—	—	0

Diazepam, zopiclone, Buscopan and Lomotil – as in Method 1.
Notes: The lofexidine and symptomatic medication courses run concurrently. As with Method 1, the total supply may be divided into two prescriptions.

Method 3 – Dihydrocodeine plus symptomatic medication

Dihydrocodeine (30 mg tablets)

Take medication in divided doses four times a day, with 4 to 6 hours between doses. The following are the *maximum* daily doses.

Day	No. of tablets
1	12
2	18
3	20
4	20
5	20
6	18

7	16
may start here, see note	
8	14
9	12
10	10
start symptomatic medication here	
11	8
12	6
13	4
14	2

Diazepam, zopiclone, Buscopan and Lomotil – as in Method 1, or smaller amounts may be adequate

Notes: In this method the medication supply is always divided into a series of prescriptions, each for 3 to 4 days' supply.

The symptomatic medication only begins 4 days from the end of the dihydrocodeine course, as indicated.

Not all patients require the relatively high dihydrocodeine doses suggested at the start of the course. If this method is used to detoxify from low levels of heroin, a shorter course may be used, as indicated. Some adjustments may be necessary to have the maximum dihydrocodeine dose about 3 days into the detoxification.

Glossary

This explains some of the terms which are used in the book. Drugs slang is not included, as this varies greatly between countries and local areas.

Addictiveness	Propensity of a drug to cause dependence, particularly withdrawal symptoms
Agonist	A drug which produces a specified chemical action
Amphetamine	Stimulant drug, often in the form of an impure powder or a paste, as 'base'
Ampoule	Glass phial of a pharmaceutical drug
Antagonist	A drug which produces the opposite of a specified chemical action
Barbiturates	Tranquillizers commonly used before the benzodiazepines were introduced – Tuinal, Seconal, etc.
Benzodiazepines	Widely prescribed tranquillizers – diazepam, nitrazepam, etc.
Buprenorphine	Medication with both opioid agonist and antagonist actions
Cannabis	Herbal sedative drug, with various forms derived from different parts of the plant
Cocaine	Stimulant drug, has typically been relatively expensive. The powder form is cocaine hydrochloride, but increasingly the more potent *crack* is used, in the form of crystalline 'rocks'
Community treatment	Treatment in which individuals are managed in or near their own home, often in liaison with other local agencies
Cyclizine	Antiemetic medication, tablets of which are abused by injection
Dependence	State in which there is a strong requirement for a drug, particularly characterized by varying degrees of tolerance, craving and withdrawal symptoms. If withdrawal symptoms are of a bodily kind, e.g. tremor or fits, the term *physical dependence* can be used
Detoxification	The process of controlled withdrawal from a drug
Dextromoramide	(Palfium) Opioid medication, frequently abused by injection
Diamorphine	Heroin – the chemical term diamorphine may be used to refer to the pharmaceutical preparation
Dipipanone	(Diconal) Opioid medication, highly regarded by drug misusers
Dual diagnosis	Strictly speaking, refers to any combination of psychiatric (or other) diagnoses, but increasingly used to indicate substance misuse plus a psychiatric condition, e.g. schizophrenia, depression
Ecstasy	Methylenedioxymethamphetamine – a stimulant drug with additional semihallucinogenic effects

Hard drugs	A term usually discouraged by professionals, but which can be used to refer to the more addictive drugs
Harm reduction	A range of policy measures aimed at reducing the harm which comes from drug misuse, rather than eliminating it completely
Heroin	Highly addictive sedative drug, usually in the form of an impure powder
HIV	Human Immunodeficiency Virus, which exists in different forms. Also refers to the fatal disease caused by the virus, AIDS
HIV-risk behaviours	Behaviours which increase the risk of acquiring or transmitting HIV, including various injecting and sexual practices
Illicit drugs	Drugs which are illegal to obtain or use in a specific country
Injectable medication	Usually refers to preparations which are meant to be injected, e.g. methadone ampoules, although can refer to tablets, etc., which may be abused by injection
LAAM	Levo-alpha-acetyl methadol. A long-acting equivalent of methadone
Lofexidine	Analogue of clonidine with fewer adverse effects, used in opiate detoxification
Low threshold treatment	Treatment – often methadone – made easy to obtain, as part of a harm-reduction approach
Maintenance	Ongoing substitution treatment, usually with methadone or buprenorphine
MDMA	Methylenedioxymethamphetamine. See ecstasy
Methadone	Synthetic opioid medication used as a so-called 'heroin substitute'
Motivation	Desire to change drug-taking behaviour or have treatment. May be enhanced by *motivational interviewing*
Naltrexone	Opioid antagonist used to block the effects of heroin or related drugs
Narcotic	Technically means sleep-inducing, but various usages refer to opiates or 'hard drugs' in general
Narcotic blockade	Effect by which methadone is claimed to nullify the actions of other opiates or opioids if taken
Opiates	Naturally occurring heroin-like drugs, including heroin itself
Opioids	Synthetic heroin-like drugs
Palfium	See dextromoramide
Primary care	The general practice treatment setting
Recreational drug use	A much derided term which refers to drug use which is relatively unproblematic and seen as a lifestyle choice
Rehabilitation	The process of learning to live without drugs. May be formally approached in a residential *rehabilitation centre*. A broader usage of the term refers to almost any treatment
Secondary service	Specialist service to which general practitioners and others may refer
Sedative drugs	('downers') Range of drugs with predominantly sedating and tranquillizing effects

Serotonin	Brain chemical which is important in determining mood and some of the effects of drugs. One group of antidepressants is the *specific serotonergic re-uptake inhibitors*
Soft drugs	See reference to hard drugs. In this distinction, soft drugs are the less addictive kinds
Solvent misuse	Problematic use, by sniffing, of glues, lighter fuels, etc. which contain various volatile substances
Stimulant drugs	('uppers') Range of drugs with predominantly stimulant and energizing effects
Substance misuse	Problematic use of any chemical substance
Substitution treatment	Treatment in which an individual receives a medication with broadly similar effects to their drug of dependence
Therapeutic community	Residential rehabilitation centre based on a particularly strong 'concept' or religious theme
Tolerance	The phenomenon whereby increasing amounts of drug are required to achieve the same effect
Twelve-step treatment	The conceptual basis of the methods adopted by Alcoholics Anonymous, Narcotics Anonymous and related organizations. It is considered that 'recovery' from addiction is achieved by addressing 12 specified steps in turn
Volatile substances	See solvent misuse
Withdrawal	This term is used to refer both to the symptoms which occur on stopping a drug and to the process of detoxification

References

Abou-Saleh MT (2007). Dual diagnosis: management within a psychosocial context. In: Day E (ed.) *Clinical Topics in Addiction*. London: RCPsych Publications, pp. 169–83

Abraham HD & Aldridge AM (1993). Adverse consequences of lysergic acid diethylamide. *Addiction*, **88**, 1327–34

Adrian M (2001). Do treatments and other interventions work? Some critical issues. *Substance Use and Misuse*, **36**, 1759–80

Advisory Council on the Misuse of Drugs (1982). *Treatment and Rehabilitation*. Her Majesty's Stationery Office, London

Advisory Council on the Misuse of Drugs (1988). *AIDS and Drug Misuse, Part 1*. Department of Health, Her Majesty's Stationery Office, London

Advisory Council on the Misuse of Drugs (1989). *AIDS and Drug Misuse, Part 2*. Department of Health, Her Majesty's Stationery Office, London.

Advisory Council on the Misuse of Drugs (1995). *Volatile Substance Abuse*. Department of Health, Her Majesty's Stationery Office, London

Akerele EO, Levin F, Nunes E, Brady R & Kleber H (2002). Effects of HIV triple therapy on methadone levels. *American Journal on Addictions*, **11**, 308–14

Al-Adwani A & Basu N (2004). Methadone and excessive sweating. *Addiction*, **99**, 259

Alford DP, Compton P & Samet JH (2006). Acute pain management for patients receiving maintenance methadone or buprenorphine therapy. *Annals of Internal Medicine*, **144**, 127–134

Al-Hebshi NN & Skaug N (2005). Khat (Catha edulis) – an updated review. *Addiction Biology*, **10**, 299–307

Amass L, Bickel WK, Higgins ST & Badger GJ (1994). Alternate-day dosing during buprenorphine treatment of opioid dependence. *Life Sciences*, **54**, 1215–28

American Psychiatric Association (2006). Treatment of patients with substance use disorders, second edition. *American Journal of Psychiatry*, **163** suppl 8, 5–82

Andreasson S, Allebeck P, Engstrom A et al. (1987). Cannabis and schizophrenia. A longitudinal study of Swedish conscripts. *The Lancet*, **ii**, 1483–6

Appel PW, Joseph H, Kott A, Nottingham W, Tasiny E & Habel E (2001). Selected in-treatment outcomes of long-term methadone maintenance treatment patients in New York State. *The Mount Sinai Journal of Medicine*, **68**, 55–61

Arendt M, Rosenberg R, Foldager L, Perto G & Minuk-Jorgensen P (2005). Cannabis-induced psychosis and subsequent schizophrenia-spectrum disorders: follow-up study of 535 incident cases. *British Journal of Psychiatry*, **187**, 510–15

Arseneault L, Cannon M, Witten J & Murray R (2004). Causal association between cannabis and psychosis: examination of the evidence. *British Journal of Psychiatry*, **184**, 110–17

Auriacombe M, Franques P, Daulouede JP & Tignol J (1999). The French experience: results from extensive delimited research studies and nation-wide sample surveys. *Research and Clinical Forums*, **21**, 9–15

Aveyard P & West R (2007). Managing smoking cessation. *British Medical Journal*, **335**, 37–41

Babor TF (2006). The diagnosis of cannabis dependence. In: Roffman RA & Stephens RS (eds.) *Cannabis Dependence: Its nature, consequences and treatment*. London: Cambridge University Press, pp. 21–36

Babor TF & Grant M (1989). From clinical research to secondary prevention: international collaboration in the development of the Alcohol Use Disorders Identification Test (AUDIT). *Alcohol Health and Research World*, **13**, 371–4

Backmund M, Meyer K, Eichenlaub D & Schütz CG (2001). Predictors for completing an inpatient detoxification program among intravenous heroin users, methadone substituted and codeine substituted patients. *Drug and Alcohol Dependence*, **64**, 173–80

Baker A, Lee NK, Claire M, Lewin TJ, Grant T, Pohlman S, Saunders JB, Kay-Lambkin F, Constable P, Jenner L & Carr VJ (2005). Brief cognitive behavioural interventions for regular amphetamine users: a step in the right direction. *Addiction*, **100**, 367–78

Ball AL (2007). HIV, injecting drug use and harm reduction: a public health response. *Addiction*, **102**, 684–90

Ball D (2008). Addiction science and its genetics. *Addiction*, **103**, 360–7

Ball SA (2007). Comparing individual therapies for personality disordered opioid dependent patients. *Journal of Personality Disorders*, **21**, 305–21

Ball JC & Ross A (1991). *The Effectiveness of Methadone Maintenance Treatment: Patients, Programs, Services and Outcome.* New York: Springer-Verlag

Ball JC & van de Wijngaart GF (1994). A Dutch addict's view of methadone maintenance – an American and a Dutch appraisal. *Addiction*, **89**, 799–802

Banbery J, Wolff K & Raistrick D (2000). Dihydrocodeine: a useful tool in the detoxification of methadone-maintained patients. *Journal of Substance Abuse Treatment*, **19**, 301–5

Bank PA & Silk KR (2001). Axis I and Axis II interactions. *Current Opinion in Psychiatry*, **14**, 137–42

Barrau K, Thirion X, Micallef J, Chuniaud-Louche C, Bellemin B, Marco S & Jean L (2001). Comparison of methadone and high dosage buprenorphine users in French care centres. *Addiction*, **96**, 1433–41

Bartels SJ, Drake RE, Wallach MA et al. (1991). Characteristic hostility in schizophrenic outpatients. *Schizophrenia Bulletin*, **17**, 163–71

Bartholomew NG & Rowan-Szal GA (2002). Sexual abuse among women entering methadone treatment. *Journal of Psychoactive Drugs*, **34**, 347–54

Bartu A, Freeman NC, Gawthorne GS, Allsop SJ & Quigley AJ (2002). Characteristics, retention and readmissions of opioid-dependent clients treated with oral naltrexone. *Drug & Alcohol Review*, **21**, 335–40

Baylen CA & Rosenberg H (2006). A review of the acute subjective effects of MDMA/ecstasy. *Addiction*, **101**, 933–47

Beaini AY, Johnson TS, Langstaffe P, Carr MP, Crossfield JN & Sweeney RC (2000). A compressed opiate detoxification regime with naltrexone maintenance: patient tolerance, risk assessment and abstinence rates. *Addiction Biology*, **5**, 451–62

Bearn J, Gossop M & Strang J (1996). Randomised double-blind comparison of lofexidine and methadone in the inpatient treatment of opiate withdrawal. *Drug and Alcohol Dependence*, **43**, 87–91

Bell J, Bowron P, Lewis J & Batey R (1990). Serum levels of methadone in maintenance clients who persist in illicit drug use. *British Journal of Addiction*, **85**, 1599–602

Bell J, Dru A, Fischer B, Levit S & Sarfraz MA (2002). Substitution therapy for heroin addiction. *Substance Use and Misuse*, **37**, 1149–78

Ben Amar M & Potvin S (2007). Cannabis and psychosis: what is the link? *Journal of Psychoactive Drugs*, **39**, 131–142

Bennett GA, Davies E & Thomas P (2003). Is oral fluid analysis as accurate as urinalysis in detecting drug use in a treatment setting? *Drug and Alcohol Dependence*, **72**, 265–9

Bertschy G (1995). Methadone maintenance treatment: an update. *European Archives of Psychiatry and Clinical Neuroscience*, **245**, 114–24

Best D, Noble A, Man LH, Gossop M, Finch E & Strang J (2002). Factors surrounding long-term benzodiazepine prescribing in methadone maintenance clients. *Journal of Substance Abuse Treatment*, **7**, 175–9

Beswick T, Best D, Rees S, Bearn J, Gossop M & Strang J (2003). Major disruptions of sleep during treatment of the opiate withdrawal syndrome: differences between methadone and lofexidine detoxification treatments. *Addiction Biology*, **8**, 49–57

Bickel WK & Amass L (1995). Buprenorphine treatment of opioid dependence: a review. *Experimental and Clinical Psychopharmacology*, **3**, 477–89

Bigwood CS & Coehelho AJ (1990). Methadone and caries. *British Dental Journal*, **168**, 231

Bird SM & Hutchinson SJ (2003). Male drugs-related deaths in the fortnight after release from prison: Scotland, 1996–99. *Addiction*, **98**, 185–190

Bluhm EC, Daniels J, Pollock BH, Olshan AF, Children's Oncology Group (United States) (2006). Maternal use of recreational drugs and neuroblastoma in offspring: a report from the Children's Oncology Group (United States). *Cancer Causes & Control*, 17, 663–9

Bond A (1993). The risks of taking benzodiazepines. In: Hallstrom C (ed.) *Benzodiazepine Dependence*. Oxford: Oxford Medical Publications, pp. 34–45

Boutros NN & Bowers MB Jnr (1996). Chronic substance-induced psychotic disorders: state of the literature. *Journal of Neuropsychiatry and Clinical Neuroscience*, 8, 262–9

Bowden-Jones O, Iqbal MZ, Tyrer P, Seivewright N, Cooper S, Judd A & Weaver T (2004). Prevalence of personality disorder in alcohol and drug services and associated comorbidity. *Addiction*, 99, 1306–14

Boys A, Lenton S & Norcross K (1997). Polydrug use at raves by a Western Australian sample. *Drug and Alcohol Review*, 16, 227–34

Bradbeer TM, Fleming PM, Charlton P & Crichton JS (1998). Survey of amphetamine prescribing in England and Wales. *Drug and Alcohol Review*, 17, 299–304

Breen CL, Harris SJ, Lintzeris N, Mattick RP, Hawken L, Bell J, Ritter AJ, Lenne M & Mendoza E (2003). Cessation of methadone maintenance treatment using buprenorphine: transfer from methadone to buprenorphine and subsequent buprenorphine reductions. *Drug and Alcohol Dependence*, 71, 49–55

Brewer C (1996). On the specific effectiveness, and under-valuing, of pharmacological treatments for addiction: a comparison of methadone, naltrexone and disulfiram with psychosocial interventions. *Addiction Research*, 3, 297–313

British National Formulary (2008). Vol 55

Broekaert E & Vanderplasschen W (2003). Towards the integration of treatment systems for substance abusers: Report on the Second International Symposium on Substance Abuse Treatment and Special Target Groups. *Journal of Psychoactive Drugs*, 35, 237–45

Brook JS, Brook DW & Pahl K (2006). The developmental context for adolescence substance abuse intervention. In: Liddle HA & Rowe CL (eds.) *Adolescent Substance Abuse: Research and Clinical Advances*. Cambridge University Press, pp. 25–51

Brooner RK, Greenfield L, Schmidt C & Bigelow GE (1993). Antisocial personality disorder and HIV infection among intravenous drug abusers. *American Journal of Psychiatry*, 150, 53–8

Brower KJ (2002). Anabolic steroid abuse and dependence. *Current Psychiatry Reports*, 4, 377–87

Brown R, Balousek S, Mundt M & Fleming M (2005). Methadone maintenance and male sexual dysfunction. *Journal of Addictive Diseases*, 24, 91–106

Brownell LW & Naik PC (2003). Services for opiate misuse: can primary care meet government expectations? *Psychiatric Bulletin*, 27, 328–30

Brugal MT, Domingo-Salvany A, Puig R, Barrio G, Garcia de Olalla P & de la Fuente L (2005). Evaluating the impact of methadone maintenance programmes on mortality due to overdose and AIDS in a cohort of heroin users in Spain. *Addiction*, 100, 981–9

Brunette MF & Drake RE (1997). Gender differences in patients with schizophrenia and substance abuse. *Comprehensive Psychiatry*, 38, 109–16

Budney AJ, Bickel WK & Amass L (1998). Marijuana use and treatment outcome among opioid-dependent patients. *Addiction*, 93, 493–503

Budney AJ, Moore B, Sigmon SC & Higgins ST (2006). Contingency-management interventions for cannabis dependence. In: Roffman RA & Stephens RS (eds.) *Cannabis Dependence: Its nature, consequences and treatment*. London: Cambridge University Press, pp. 155–66

Buning EC, van Brussel GHA, van Santen MD & van Santen G (1990). The 'methadone by bus' project in Amsterdam. *British Journal of Addiction*, 85, 1247–50

Buntwal N, Bearn J, Gossop M & Strang J (2000). Naltrexone and lofexidine combination treatment compared with conventional lofexidine treatment for in-patient opiate detoxification. *Drug and Alcohol Dependence*, 59, 183–8

Burmeister JJ, Lungren EM & Neisewander JL (2003). Effects of fluoxetine and d-fenfluramine on cocaine-seeking behavior in rats. *Psychopharmacology*, 168, 146–54

Burns L, Mattick RP, Lim K & Wallace C (2006). Methadone in pregnancy: treatment retention and neonatal outcomes. *Addiction*, 102, 264–70

Calsyn DA, Malcy JA & Saxon AJ (2006). Slow tapering from methadone maintenance in a program encouraging indefinite mainten-ance. *Journal of Substance Abuse Treatment*, **30**, 159–63

Calsyn DA, Wells EA, Fleming C & Saxon AJ (2000). Changes in Millon Clinical Multiaxial Inventory scores among opiate addicts as a function of retention in methadone mainten-ance treatment and recent drug use. *American Journal of Drug and Alcohol Abuse*, **26**, 297–309

Canagasaby A & Vinson DC (2005). Screening for hazardous or harmful drinking using one or two quantity-frequency questions. *Alcohol & Alcoholism*, **40**, 208–13

Capelhorn JRM (1994). A comparison of abstinence-oriented and indefinite metha-done maintenance treatment. *International Journal of the Addictions*, **29**, 1361–75

Capelhorn JRM & Ross MW (1995). Methadone maintenance and the likelihood of risky needle-sharing. *International Journal of the Addictions*, **30**, 685–98

Carnwath T & Merrill J (2002). Dose equivalents in opioid substitution treatment. *Inter-national Journal of Drug Policy*, **13**, 445–7

Carnwath T & Smith I (2002). *Heroin Century*. London: Routledge

Carnwath T, Gabbay M & Barnard J (2000). A share of the action: general practitioner involvement in drug misuse treatment in Greater Manchester. *Drugs; Education, Pre-vention and Policy*, 7, 235–44

Carnwath T, Garvey T & Holland M (2002). The prescription of dexamphetamine to patients with schizophrenia and amphetamine dependence. *Journal of Psychopharmacology*, **16**, 372–7

Carpenter KM, Brooks AC, Vosburg SK & Nunes EV (2004). The effect of sertraline and environmental context on treating depression and illicit substance use among methadone maintained opiate dependent patients: a controlled clinical trial. *Drug and Alcohol Dependence*, **74**, 123–34

Carreno JE, Alvarez CE, San Narciso GI, Bascaran MT, Diaz M & Bobes J (2003). Maintenance treatment with depot opioid antagonists in subcutaneous implants: an alternative in the treatment of opioid dependence. *Addiction Biology*, **8**, 429–38

Carrieri MP, Amass L, Lucas GM, Vlahov D, Wodak A & Woody GE (2006). Buprenor-phine use: the international experience. *Clinical Infectious Diseases*, **43**, S197–215

Castells X, Casas M, Vildal X, Bosch R, Roncero C, Ramos-Quiroga JA & Capella D (2007) Effi-cacy of central nervous system stimulant treatment for cocaine dependence: a systematic review and meta-analysis of randomized con-trolled clinical trials. *Addiction*, **102**, 1871–87

Chaisson RE, Bacchetti P, Osmond D, Brodie B, Sande MA & Moss AR (1989). Cocaine use and HIV infection in intravenous drug users in San Francisco. *Journal of the American Medical Association*, **261**, 561–5

Chapleo CB & Walter DS (1997). The bupre-norphine–naloxone combination product. *Research and Clinical Forums*, **19**, 55–8

Cheskin LJ, Fudala PJ & Johnson RE (1994). A controlled comparison of buprenorphine and clonidine for acute detoxification from opioids. *Drug and Alcohol Dependence*, **36**, 115–21

Coffin PO, Galea S, Ahern J, Leon AC, Vlahov D & Tardiff K (2003). Opiates, cocaine and alcohol combinations in accidental drug overdose deaths in New York City. *Addic-tion*, **98**, 739–47

Colado MI, O'Shea E & Green AR (2004). Acute and long-term effects of MDMA on cerebral dopamine biochemistry and function. *Psy-chopharmacology*, **173**, 249–63

Cole JC & Sumnall HR (2003). Altered states: The clinical effects of ecstasy. *Pharmacology and Therapeutics*, **98**, 35–58

Conklin CA & Tiffany ST (2002). Applying extinction research and theory to cue-exposure addiction treatments. *Addiction*, **97**, 155–67

Connell PH (1958). *Amphetamine Psychosis*. Institute of Psychiatry Maudsley Monograph No. 5. London; Oxford University Press

Conner KR, Pinquart M & Duberstein PR (2008). Meta-analysis of depression and substance use and impairment among intravenous drug users (IDUs). *Addiction*, **103**, 524–34

Conrod PJ, Stewart SH, Pihl RO, Cote S, Fon-taine V & Dongier M (2000). Efficacy of brief coping skills interventions that match different personality profiles of female sub-stance abusers. *Psychology of Addictive Behaviors*, **14**, 231–42

Corkery JM, Schifano F, Ghodse AH & Oyefeso A (2004). The effects of methadone and its role in fatalities. *Human Psychopharmacol-ogy*, **19**, 565–76

Covi L, Hess JM, Kreiter NA & Haertzen CA (1995). Effects of combined fluoxetine and counselling in the outpatient treatment of cocaine abusers. *American Journal of Drug & Alcohol Abuse*, **21**, 327–44

Craig RJ, Olson R & Shalton G (1990). Improvement in psychological functioning among drug abusers: inpatient treatment compared to outpatient methadone maintenance. *Journal of Substance Abuse Treatment*, **7**, 11–19

Crits-Christoph P, Siqueland L, Blaine J et al. (1999). Psychosocial treatments for cocaine dependence: National Institute on Drugs Abuse collaborative cocaine treatment study. *Archives of General Psychiatry*, **56**, 493–502

Crofts N, Nigro L, Oman K, Stevenson G & Sherman J (1997). Methadone maintenance and hepatitis C virus infection among injecting drug users. *Addiction*, **92**, 999–1005

Crome IB & Myton T (2007). Pharmacotherapy in dual diagnosis. In: Day E (ed.) *Clinical Topics in Addiction*. London: RCPsych Publications, pp. 149–68

Cuffel BJ, Shumway M, Chouljian TL et al. (1994). A longitudinal study of substance use and community violence in schizophrenia. *Journal of Nervous and Mental Disease*, **182**, 704–8

Curran C, Byrappa N & McBride A (2004). Stimulant psychosis: systematic review. *British Journal of Psychiatry*, **185**, 196–204

Dallery J, Silverman K, Chutuape MA, Bigelow GE & Stitzer ML (2001). Voucher-based reinforcement of opiate plus cocaine abstinence in treatment-resistant methadone patients: effects of reinforcer magnitude. *Experimental and Clinical Psychopharmacology*, **9**, 317–25

Darke S (1998). The effectiveness of methadone maintenance treatment. 3: Moderators of treatment outcome. In: Ward J, Mattick RP, Hall W (eds.) *Methadone Maintenance Treatment and Other Opioid Replacement Therapies*. London: Harwood, pp. 75–90

Darke S, Hall W, Wodak A, Heather N & Ward J (1992a). Development and validation of a multi-dimensional instrument for assessing outcome of treatment among opiate users: the Opiate Treatment Index. *British Journal of Addiction*, **87**, 733–42

Darke S, Hall W, Ross MW & Wodak A (1992b). Benzodiazepine use and HIV risk-taking behaviour among injecting drug users. *Drug and Alcohol Dependence*, **31**, 31–6

Darke S, Swift W, Hall W & Ross M (1993). Drug use, HIV risk-taking and psychosocial correlates of benzodiazepine use among methadone maintenance clients. *Drug and Alcohol Dependence*, **34**, 67–70

Darke S, Ross J & Cohen J (1994a). The use of benzodiazepines among regular amphetamine users. *Addiction*, **89**, 1683–90

Darke S, Hall W & Swift W (1994b). Prevalence, symptoms and correlates of antisocial personality disorder among methadone maintenance clients. *Drug and Alcohol Dependence*, **34**, 253–7

Darke S, Sims J, McDonald S & Wickes W (2000). Cognitive impairment among methadone maintenance patients. *Addiction*, **95**, 687–95

Darke S, Topp L & Ross J (2002). The injection of methadone and benzodiazepines among Sydney injecting drug users 1996–2000: 5-year monitoring of trends from the Illicit Drug Reporting System. *Drug and Alcohol Review*, **21**, 27–32

Darke S, Ross J, Teesson M & Lynskey M (2003). Health service utilization and benzodiazepine use among heroin users: findings from the Australian Treatment Outcome Study (ATOS). *Addiction*, **98**, 1129–35

Darke S, Ross J, Williamson A, Mills KL, Harvard A & Teesson M (2007). Borderline personality disorder and persistently elevated levels of risk in 36 month outcomes for the treatment of heroin dependence. *Addiction*, **102**, 1140–6

Dawe S, Griffiths P, Gossop M & Strang J (1991). Should opiate addicts be involved in controlling their own detoxification? A comparison of fixed versus negotiable schedules. *British Journal of Addiction*, **86**, 977–82

Day E & George S (2007). *Management of drug misuse in pregnancy.* In: Day E (ed.) *Clinical Topics in Addiction*, London: RCPsych Publications, pp. 259–74

Day E, Porter L, Clarke A, Allen D, Moselhy H & Copello A (2003). Drug misuse in pregnancy: the impact of a specialist treatment service. *Psychiatric Bulletin*, **27**, 99–101

De Leon G, Staines GL & Sacks S (1997). Passages: a therapeutic community oriented day treatment model for methadone maintained clients. *Journal of Drug Issues*, **27**, 341–66 de Lima MS, de Oliveira Soares BG, Reisser AAP & Farrell M (2002). Pharmacological treatment of cocaine dependence: a systematic review. *Addiction*, **97**, 931–49

Deltsidou A (2001). Cocaine abuse in pregnancy. *Review of Clinical Pharmacology and Pharmacokinetics International Edition*, **15**, suppl 225–32

Department of Health (1991). *Drug Misuse and Dependence: Guidelines on Clinical Management*. London: HMSO

Department of Health (1999). *Drug Misuse and Dependence: Guidelines on Clinical Management*. London: HMSO

Department of Health (2007). *Drug Misuse and Dependence: UK Guidelines on Clinical Management*. London: DH Publications

Dey P, Roaf E, Collins S, Shaw H, Steele R & Donmall M (2002). Randomized controlled trial to assesss the effectiveness of a primary health care liaison worker in promoting shared care for opiate users. *Journal of Public Health Medicine*, **24**, 38–42

Dickey B, Normand SL, Weiss RD, Drake RE & Azeni H (2000). Medical morbidity, mental illness, and substance disorders. *Psychiatric Services*, **53**, 861–7

Dijkgraaf M, van der Zanden B, de Borgie C, Blanken P, Van Ree J & Van den Brink W (2005). Cost utility analysis of co-prescribed heroin compared with methadone maintenance treatment in heroin addicts in two randomized trials. *British Medical Journal*, **330**, 1297

Dolan K, Rutter S & Wodak AD (2003). Prison-based syringe exchange programmes: a review of international research and development. *Addiction*, **98**, 153–8

Dolan KA, Shearer J, White B, Zhou J, Kaldor J & Wodak AD (2005). Four-year follow-up of imprisoned male heroin users and methadone treatment: mortality, re-incarceration and hepatitis C infection. *Addiction*, **100**, 820–8

Dole VP (1973). Detoxification of methadone patients and public policy. *Journal of the American Medical Association*, **226**, 747–52

Dole VP (1988). Implications of methadone maintenance for theories of narcotic addiction. *Journal of the American Medical Association*, **260**, 3025–9

Dole VP & Nyswander M (1965). A medical treatment for diacetylmorphine (heroin) addiction. *Journal of the American Medical Association*, **193**, 80–84

Dole VP, Nyswander M & Kreek MJ (1966). Narcotic blockade. *Archives of Internal Medicine*, **118**, 304–9

Dole VP, Robinson JW, Orraca J, Towns E, Searcy P & Caine E (1969). Methadone treatment of randomly selected criminal addicts. *New England Journal of Medicine*, **280**, 1372–5

Donny EC, Walsh SL, Bigelow GE, Eissenberg T & Stitzer ML (2002). High-dose methadone produces superior opioid blockade and comparable withdrawal suppression to lower doses in opioid-dependent humans. *Psychopharmacology*, **161**, 202–12

Donny EC, Brasser SM, Bigelow GE, Stitzer ML & Walsh SL (2005). Methadone doses of 100 mg or greater are more effective than lower doses at suppressing heroin self-administration in opioid-dependent volunteers. *Addiction*, **100**, 1496–1509

Donovan JL, DeVane CL, Malcolm RJ, Mojsiak J, Nora-Chiang C, Elkashef A & Taylor RM (2005). Modafinil influences the pharmacokinetics of intravenous cocaine in healthy cocaine-dependent volunteers. *Clinical Pharmacokinetics*, **44**, 753–65

Drake RE, Bartels SJ, Teagues GB, Noordsy DL & Clark RE (1993). Treatment of substance abuse in severely mentally ill patients. *Journal of Nervous and Mental Disease*, **181**, 606–11

Drake RE, Mueser KT, Clark RE et al. (1996). The course, treatment and outcome of substance disorder in persons with severe mental illness. *American Journal of Orthopsychiatry*, **66**, 42–51

Drake RE, Essock SM & Shaner A (2001). Implementing dual diagnosis services for clients with severe mental illness. *Psychiatric Services*, **57**, 469–76

Drake RE, Mueser KT & Brunette MF (2007). Management of persons with co-occurring severe mental illness and substance use disorder: program implications. *World Psychiatry*, **6**, 131–6

Drummond DC, Turkington D, Rahman MZ, Mullin PJ & Jackson P (1989). Chlordiazepoxide versus methadone in opiate withdrawal: a preliminary double blind trial. *Drug and Alcohol Dependence*, **23**, 63–71

Dunn C, Deroo L & Rivara FP (2001). The use of brief interventions adapted from motivational interviewing across behavioral domains: a systematic review. *Addiction*, **96**, 1725–42

Eap CB, Buclin T & Baumann P (2002). Inter-individual variability of the clinical pharmacokinetics of methadone: implications for the treatment of opioid dependence. *Clinical Pharmacokinetics*, **41**, 1153–93

Eder H, Jagsch R, Kraigr D, Primorac A, Ebner N & Ficher G (2005). Comparative study of the effectiveness of slow-release morphine and methadone for opioid maintenance therapy. *Addiction*, **100**, 1101–9

Edwards G & Gross MM (1976). Alcohol dependence: provisional description of a clinical syndrome. *British Medical Journal*, **1**, 1058–61

Edwards G, Marshall EJ & Cook CCH (2003). *The Treatment of Drinking Problems: A Guide for the Helping Professions*, 4th ed. Cambridge: Cambridge University Press

Eissenberg T, Bigelow GE, Strain EC, Walsh SL, Brooner RK, Stitzer ML & Johnson RE (1997). Dose-related efficacy of levomethadyl acetate for treatment of opioid dependence. *Journal of the American Medical Association*, **277**, 1945–51

Eklund C, Melin L, Hiltunen A & Borg S (1994). Detoxification from methadone maintenance treatment in Sweden: long-term outcome and effects on quality of life and life situation. *The International Journal of the Addictions*, **29**, 627–45

el-Guebaly N (2004). Concurrent substance-related disorders and mental illness: the North American experience. *World Psychiatry*, **3**, 182–7

Epstein DH & Preston KL (2003). Does cannabis use predict poor outcome for heroin-dependent patients on maintenance treatment? A review of past findings, and more evidence against. *Addiction*, **98**, 269–79

European Agency for the Evaluation of Medicinal Products (2001). http://www.emea.europa.eu/pdfs/human/press/pus/877601en.pdf

Evren C, Barut T, Saatcioglu O & Cakmak D (2006). Axis I psychiatric comorbidity among adult inhalant dependents seeking treatment. *Journal of Psychoactive Drugs*, **38**, 57–64

Faggiano F, Vigna-Taglianti F & Lemma P (2004). Methadone maintenance at different dosages for opioid dependence. *The Cochrane Library*, Issue 2. Chichester, UK: Wiley

Fajemirokun-Odudeyi O & Lindow SW (2004). Obstetric implications of cocaine use in pregnancy: a literature review. *European Journal of Obstetrics and Gynecology and Reproductive Biology*, **112**, 2–8

Falck R, Wang J & Carlson RG (2007). Crack cocaine trajectories among users in a midwestern American city. *Addiction*, **102**, 1421–31

Fals-Stewart W, O'Farrell TJ & Birchler GR (2001). Behavioral couples therapy for male methadone maintenance patients: effects on drug-using behaviour relationship adjustment. *Behaviour Therapy*, **32**, 391–411

Farre M, Mas A, Torrens M, Moreno V & Cami J (2002). Retention rate and illicit opioid use during methadone maintenance interventions: a meta-analysis. *Drug & Alcohol Dependence*, **65**, 283–90

Farrell M & Marsden J (2008). Acute risk of drug-related death among newly released prisoners in England and Wales. *Addiction*, **103**, 251–5

Farrell M, Battersby M & Strang J (1990). Screening for hepatitis B and vaccination of injecting drug users in NHS drug treatment services. *British Journal of Addiction*, **85**, 1657–9

Farrell M, Neeleman J, Griffiths P & Strang J (1996). Suicide and overdose among opiate addicts. *Addiction*, **91**, 321–3

Farrell M, Howes S, Bebbington P, Brugha T, Jenkins R, Lewis G, Marsden J, Taylor C & Meltzer H (2001). Nicotine, alcohol and drug dependence and psychiatric comorbidity. *British Journal of Psychiatry*, **179**, 432–7

Farrell M, Gowing L, Marsden J et al. (2005). Effectiveness of drug dependence treatment in HIV prevention. *International Journal of Drug Policy*, **16**, supp l67–75

Farren CK (1997). The use of naltrexone, an opiate antagonist, in the treatment of opiate addiction. *Irish Journal of Psychological Medicine*, **14**, 26–31

Fatseas M, Lavie E, Denis C, Franques RP & Tignol J (2006). Benzodiazepine withdrawal in subjects on opiate substitution treatment. *Presse Medicale*, **35**, 599–606

Federman EB, Costello EJ, Angold A, Farmer EMZ & Erkanli A (1997). Development of substance use and psychiatric comorbidity in an epidemiologic study of white and

American Indian young adolescents. The Great Smoky Mountains Study. *Drug and Alcohol Dependence*, **44**, 69–78

Feeney GFX, Connor JP, Young RMcD, Tucker J & McPherson A (2006). Improvement in measures of psychological distresss amongst amphetamine misusers treated with brief cognitive-behavioural therapy (CBT). *Addictive Behaviors*, **31**, 1833–43

Felice AM & Kouimtsidis C (2008). Shared care for treatment of opioid dependence and the new General Medical Services contract. *Psychiatric Bulletin*, **32**, 88–90

Fergusson DM, Poulton R, Smith TF & Boden JM (2006). Cannabis and psychosis. *British Medical Journal*, **332**, 172–5

Fiander M et al. (2003). Assertive community treatment across the Atlantic: comparison of model fidelity in the UK and USA. *British Journal of Psychiatry*, **182**, 248–54

Fiore MC, Smith SS, Jorenby DE & Baker TB (1994). The effectiveness of the nicotine patch for smoking cessation: a meta-analysis. *Journal of the American Medical Association*, **271**, 1940–7

Fiorentine R & Anglin MD (1996). More is better: counselling participation and the effectiveness of outpatient drug treatment. *Journal of Substance Abuse and Treatment*, **13**, 341–8

Fischer G (2000). Treatment of opioid dependence in pregnant women. *Addiction*, **102**, 264–70

Fischer G, Presslich O, Diamant K, Schneider C, Pezawas L & Kasper S (1996). Oral morphine-sulphate in the treatment of opiate dependent patients. *Alcoholism*, **32**, 35–43

Fischer GW, Johnson RE, Eder H et al. (2000). Treatment of opioid-dependent pregnant women with buprenorphine. *Addiction*, **95**, 239–44

Flaum M & Schultz SK (1996). When does amphetamine-induced psychosis become schizophrenia? *American Journal of Psychiatry*, **153**, 812–5

Fleming PM & Roberts D (1994). Is the prescription of amphetamine justified as a harm reduction measure? *Journal of the Royal Society of Health*, June, 127–30

Fleming ME, Mundt MP, French MT, Manwell LB, Staauffacher EA & Barry KL (2002). Brief physician advice for problem drinkers: long-term efficacy and cost-benefit analysis. *Alcoholism Clinical Experimental Research*, **26**, 36–43

Flynn PM, Joe GW, Broome KM, Simpson DD & Brown BS (2003). Recovery from opioid addiction in DATOS. *Journal of Substance Abuse Treatment*, **25**, 177–86

Foltin RW & Fischman MW (1996). Effects of methadone or buprenorphine maintenance on the subjective and reinforcing effects of intravenous cocaine in humans. *Journal of Pharmacology and Experimental Therapeutics*, **278**, 1153–64

Fowler T, Lifford K, Shelton K, Rice F, Thapar A, Neale MC, McBride A & van den Bree BM (2007). Exploring the relationship between genetic and environmental influences on initiation and progression of substance use. *Addiction*, **101**, 413–22

Fugelstad A, Stenbacka M, Leifman A, Nylander M & Thiblin I (2007). Methadone maintenance treatment: the balance between life-saving treatment and fatal poisonings. *Addiction*, **102**, 406–12

Galanter M, Egelko S, De Leon G, Rohrs C & Franco H (1992). Crack cocaine abusers in the general hospital: assessment and initiation of care. *American Journal of Psychiatry*, **149**, 810–15

Galanter M, Egelko S, Edwards H & Vergaray M (1994). A treatment system for combined psychiatric and addictive illness. *Addiction*, **89**, 1227–35

Gawin FH & Kleber HD (1986). Abstinence symptomatology and psychiatric diagnoses in cocaine abusers: clinical observations. *Archives of General Psychiatry*, **43**, 107–13

Gazzard B, Anderson J, Babiker A et al. (2005). British HIV Association (BHIVA) guidelines for the treatment of HIV-infected adults with antiretroviral therapy (2005). *HIV Medicine*, **6**, suppl 2, 1–61

George S & Braithwaite RA (2000). Using amphetamine isomer ratios to determine the compliance of amphetamine abusers prescribed Dexedrine. *Journal of Analytical Toxicology*, **24**, 223–7

Gerada C & Limber C (2003). General practitioners with special interests: implications for clinical governance. *Quality in Primary Care*, **11**, 47–52

Gerra G, Marcato A, Caccavari R et al. (1995). Clonidine and opiate receptor antagonists in the treatment of heroin addiction. *Journal of Substance Abuse Treatment*, **12**, 35–41.

Gerra G, Zaimovic A, Giusti F, Di Gennaro C, Zambelli U, Gardini S & Delsignore R (2001). Lofexidine versus clonidine in rapid opiate detoxification. *Journal of Substance Abuse Treatment*, **21**, 11–7

Gerra G, Ferri M, Polidori E, Santoro G, Zaimovic A & Sternieri E (2003). Long-term methadone maintenance effectiveness: psychosocial and pharmacological variables. *Journal of Substance Abuse Treatment*, **25**, 1–8

Ghodse H (2007). 'Uppers' keep going up. *British Journal of Psychiatry*, **191**, 279–81

Giacomuzzi SM, Riemer Y, Ertl M, Kemmler H, Rössler H, Hinterhuber H & Kurz M (2003). Buprenorphine versus methadone maintenance treatment in an ambulant setting: a health-related quality of life assessment. *Addiction*, **98**, 693–702

Gibson DR, Flynn NM & McCarthy JJ (1999). Effectiveness of methadone treatment in reducing HIV risk behaviour and HIV seroconversion among injecting drug users. *AIDS*, **13**, 1807–18

Gilvarry E & Crome IB (2004). Implications of parental substance misuse. In: Crome I, Ghodse H, Gilvarry E and McArdle P (eds.) *Young People and Substance Misuse*. London: Gaskell Publications, pp. 85–100

Gill K, Nolimal D & Crowley TJ (1992). Antisocial personality disorder, HIV risk behaviour and retention in methadone maintenance therapy. *Drug and Alcohol Dependence*, **30**, 247–52

Gilman SM, Galanter M & Dermatis H (2001). Methadone Anonymous: a 12-step program for methadone maintained heroin addicts. *Substance Abuse*, **22**, 247–56

Glasper A, Reed LJ, De Wet CJ, Gossop M & Bearn J (2005). Induction of patients with moderately severe methadone dependence onto buprenorphine. *Addiction Biology*, **10**, 149–55

Gold MS (1993). Opiate addiction and the locus coeruleus. *Psychiatric Clinics of North America*, **16**, 61–73

Goldstein A & Brown BW (2003). Urine testing in methadone maintenance treatment: applications and limitations. *Journal of Substance Abuse Treatment*, **25**, 61–3

Gonzalez JP & Brogden RN (1988). Naltrexone: a review of its pharmacodynamic and pharmacokinetic properties and therapeutic efficacy in the management of opioid dependence. *Drugs*, **35**, 192–213

Gossop M & Moos R (2008). Substance misuse among older adults: a neglected but treatable problem. *Addiction*, **103**, 347–8

Gossop M & Strang J (1991). A comparison of the withdrawal responses of heroin and methadone addicts during detoxification. *British Journal of Psychiatry*, **158**, 697–9

Gossop M, Johns A & Green L (1986). Opiate withdrawal: inpatient versus outpatient programmes and preferred versus random assignment to treatment. *British Medical Journal*, **293**, 103–4

Gossop M, Bradley M & Philips G (1987). An investigation of withdrawal symptoms shown by opiate addicts during and subsequent to a 21–day inpatient methadone detoxification. *Addictive Behaviours*, **12**, 1–6

Gossop M, Griffiths P, Bradley M & Strang J (1989). Opiate withdrawal symptoms in response to 10–day and 21–day methadone withdrawal programmes. *British Journal of Psychiatry*, **154**, 360–3

Gossop M, Battersby M & Strang J (1991). Self-detoxification by opiate addicts: a preliminary investigation. *British Journal of Psychiatry*, **159**, 208–12

Gossop M, Marsden J, Stewart D, Lehmann P, Edwards C, Wilson A & Segar G (1998). Substance use, health and social problems of service users at 54 drug treatment agencies: intake data from the National Treatment Outcome Research Study. *British Journal of Psychiatry*, **173**, 166–71

Gossop M, Marsden J, Stewart D & Rolfe A (2000). Patterns of improvement after methadone treatment: One year follow-up results from the National Treatment Outcome Research Study (NTORS). *Drug and Alcohol Dependence*, **60**, 275–86

Gossop M, Marsden J, Stewart D & Treacy S (2001). Outcomes after methadone maintenance and methadone reduction treatments: two-year follow-up results from the National Treatment Outcome Research Study. *Drug and Alcohol Dependence*, **62**, 255–64

Gossop M, Marsden J, Stewart D & Kidd T (2002a). Changes in use of crack cocaine after drug misuse treatment: 4–5 year follow-up results from the National Treatment Outcome Research Study (NTORS). *Drug and Alcohol Dependence*, **66**, 21–8

Gossop M, Marsden J, Stewart D & Tracey S (2002b). Change and stability of change after treatment of drug misuse: 2-year outcomes from the National Treatment Outcome Research Study (UK). *Addictive Behaviors*, **27**, 155–66

Gossop M, Marsden J, Stewart D & Kidd T (2003). The National Treatment Outcome Research Study (NTORS): 4–5 year follow-up results. *Addiction*, **98**, 291–303

Gossop M, Stewart D & Marsden J (2006). Effectiveness of drugs and alcohol counselling during methadone treatment: content, frequency, and duration of counselling and association with substance use outcomes. *Addiction*, **101**, 404–12

Gossop M, Stewart D & Marsden J (2008). Attendance at Narcotics Anonymous and Alcoholics Anonymous meetings, frequency of attendance and substance use outcomes after residential treatment for drug dependence: a 5-year follow-up study. *Addiction*, **103**, 119–25

Gouzoulis-Mayfrank E & Daumann J (2006). Neurotoxicity of methylenedioxyamphetamines (MDMA; ecstasy) in humans: how strong is the evidence for persistent brain damage? *Addiction*, **101**, 348–61

Gowing L, Ali R & White J (2004). Buprenorphine for the management of opioid withdrawal (Cochrane Review). *The Cochrane Library*, Issue 2. Chichester, UK: Wiley

Gowing LR, Farrell M, Bornemann R, Sullivan LE & Ali RL (2006). Methadone treatment of injecting opioid users for prevention of HIV infection. *Journal of General Internal Medicine*, **21**, 193–5

Grabowski J, Rhodes H, Elk R, Schmitz J, Davis C, Creson D & Kirby K (1995). Fluoxetine is ineffective for treatment of cocaine dependence or concurrent opiate and cocaine dependence: two placebo-controlled, double-blind trials. *Journal of Clinical Psychopharmacology*, **15**, 163–74

Grabowski J, Rhoades H, Schmitz J, Stotts A, Daruzska LA, Creson D et al. (2001). Dextroamphetamine for cocaine-dependence treatment: a double-blind randomized clinical trial. *Journal of Clinical Psychopharmacology*, **21**, 522–6

Grabowski J, Rhoades H, Stotts A, Cowan K, Kopecky C, Dougherty A, Moeller FG, Hassan S & Schmitz J (2004). Agonist-like or antagonist-like treatment for cocaine dependence with methadone for heroin dependence: two double-blind randomized clinical trials. *Neuropsychopharmacology*, **29**, 969–81

Graham HL, Maslin J & Copello A (2001). Drug and alcohol problems amongst individuals with severe mental health problems in an inner city area of the UK. *Social Psychiatry and Psychiatric Epidemiology*, **36**, 448–55

Graham H (1998). The role of dysfunctional beliefs in individuals who experience psychosis and use substances: implications for cognitive therapy and medication adherence. *Behavioural and Cognitive Psychotherapy*, **26**, 193–208

Grant BF, Stinson FS, Dawson, DA, Chou SP, Ruan WJ & Pickering RP (2004). Co-occurrence of 12-month alcohol and drug use disorders and personality disorders in the United States: results from the National Epidemiologic Survey on Alcohol and Related Conditions. *Archives of General Psychiatry*, **61**, 361–8

Green L & Gossop M (1988). Effects of information on the opiate withdrawal syndrome. *British Journal of Addiction*, **83**, 305–9

Green B, Young R & Kavanagh D (2005). Cannabis use and misuse prevalence among people with psychosis. *British Journal of Psychiatry*, **187**, 306–13

Greenwald MK, Johanson CE, Moody DE, Woods JH, Kilbourne MR, Koeppe RA, Schuster CR & Zubieta JK (2003). Effects of buprenorphine maintenance dose on m-opioid receptor availability, plasma concentrations, and antagonist blockade in heroin-dependent volunteers. *Neuropsychopharmacology*, **28**, 2000–9

Greenwood J (1996). Six years of sharing the care of Edinburgh drug users. *Psychiatric Bulletin*, **20**, 8–11

Grella CE, Anglin MD & Wugalter SE (1997). Patterns and predictors of cocaine and crack use by clients in standard and enhanced methadone maintenance treatment. *American Journal of Drug and Alcohol Abuse*, **23**, 15–42

Griffin ML, Weiss RD, Mirin SM, Wilson H & Bouchard-Voelk B (1987). The use of the Diagnostic Interview Schedule in drug-dependent patients. *American Journal of Drug and Alcohol Abuse*, **13**, 281–91

Griffin S, Campbell A & McCaldin H (2008). A 'dual diagnosis' community psychiatric nurse service in Lanarkshire: service innovation. *Psychiatric Bulletin*, **32**, 139–42

Gross A, Jacobs EA, Petry NM, Badger GJ & Bickel WK (2001). Limits to buprenorphine dosing: a comparison between quintuple and sextuple the maintenance dose every 5 days. *Drug & Alcohol Dependence*, **64**, 111–6

Grund JPC, Blanken P, Adriaans NFP, Kaplan CD, Barendregt C & Meenwsen M (1992). Reaching the unreached: an outreach model for 'on the spot' AIDS prevention among active, out-of-treatment drug addicts. In: O'Hare P, Newcombe R, Matthews A, Buning E & Drucker E (eds.) *The Reduction of Drug-Related Harm*. London: Routledge, pp. 172–80

Guichard A, Lert F, Calderon C et al. (2003). Illicit drug use and injections practices among drug users on methadone and buprenorphine maintenance treatment in France. *Addiction*, **98**, 1585–97

Gunne LM & Gronbladh L (1981). The Swedish methadone maintenance program: a controlled study. *Drug and Alcohol Dependence*, **7**, 249–56

Haasen C, Verthein U, Degkwitz P, Berger J, Krausz M & Naber D (2007). Heroin-assisted treatment for opioid dependence. *British Journal of Psychiatry*, **191**, 55–62

Haddock G, Barrowclough C & Tarrier N (2003). Randomised controlled trial of cognitive–behavioural therapy and motivated intervention for schizophrenia and substance use. Carer and economic outcomes at 18 months. *British Journal of Psychiatry*, **183**, 418–26

Hajak G, Müller WE, Wittchen HU, Pittrow HU & Kirch W (2003). Abuse and dependence potential for the non-benzodiazepine hypnotics zolpidem and zopiclone: a review of case reports and epidemiological data. *Addiction*, **98**, 1371–8

Halikas JA, Crosby RD, Pearson VL & Graves NM (1997). A randomised double-blind study of carbamazepine in the treatment of cocaine abuse. *Addiction of Biology*, **12**, 133–51

Hall W (2007). What's in a name? *Addiction*, **102**, 691–2

Hall W & Solowij N (1997). Long-term cannabis use and mental health. *British Journal of Psychiatry*, **171**, 107–8

Hall W & Solowij N (2006). The adverse health and psychological consequences of cannabis dependence. In: Roffman RA & Stephens RS (eds.) *Cannabis Dependence: Its nature, consequences and treatment*. Cambridge: Cambridge University Press, pp. 106–28

Hall W, Ward J & Mattick RP (1998). The effectiveness of methadone maintenance treatment 1: Heroin use and crime. In: Ward J, Mattick RP & Hall W (eds.) *Methadone Maintenance and Other Opioid Replacement Therapies*. London: Hardwood, pp. 17–58

Harrison M, Busto U, Naranjo CA, Kaplan HL & Sellers EM (1984). Diazepam tapering in detoxification for high dose benzodiazepine abuse. *Clinical Pharmacology and Therapeutics*, **36**, 527–33

Hartel DM, Schoenbaum EE, Selwyn PA, Kline J, Davenny K, Klein RS & Friedland GH (1995). Heroin use during methadone maintenance treatment: the importance of methadone dose and cocaine use. *American Journal of Public Health*, **85**, 83–8

Hartnoll RL, Mitcheson MC, Battersby A, Brown G, Ellis M, Fleming P & Hedley N (1980). Evaluation of heroin maintenance in controlled trial. *Archives of General Psychiatry*, **37**, 877–84

Harvard A, Teesson M, Darke S & Ross J (2006). Depression among heroin users: 12 month outcomes from the Australian Treatment Outcome Study (ATOS). *Journal of Substance Abuse and Treatment*, **30**, 355–62

Haugland G, Siegel C, Alexander MJ & Galanter M (1991). A survey of hospitals in New York State treating psychiatric patients with chemical abuse disorders. *Hospital and Community Psychiatry*, **42**, 1215–20

Havens JR & Strathdee SA (2005). Antisocial personality disorder and opioid treatment outcomes: a review. *Addictive Disorders and their Treatment*, **4**, 85–97

Heikkinen M, Isometsa ET, Henriksson MM, Marttunen MJ, Aro HM & Lonnqvist JK (1997). Psychosocial factors and completed suicide in personality disorders. *Acta Psychiatrica Scandinavica*, **95**, 49–57

Hellawell K (1995). The role of law enforcement in minimising the harm resulting from illicit drugs. *Drug and Alcohol Review*, **14**, 317–22

Henry JA, Jeffreys KJ & Dawling S (1992). Toxicity and deaths from 3,4–methylenedioxymethamphetamine ('ecstasy'). *The Lancet*, **340**, 384–7

Henquet C, Murray R, Linszen D & van Os J (2005). The environment and schizophrenia:

the role of cannabis use. *Schizophrenia Bulletin*, **31**, 608–12

Herve S, Riachi G, Noblet C et al. (2004). Acute hepatitis due to buprenorphine administration. *European Journal of Gastroenterology and Hepatology*, **16**, 1033–7

Higgins ST, Wong CJ, Badger GJ, Ogden DE & Dantona RL (2000). Contingent reinforcement increases cocaine abstinence during outpatient treatment and 1 year of follow-up. *Journal of Consulting and Clinical Psychology*, **68**, 64–72

Hiltunen A & Eklund C (2002). Withdrawal from methadone maintenance treatment. Reasons for not trying to quit methadone. *European Addiction Research*, **8**, 38–44

Hope VD, Judd A & Hickman M (2002). Prevalence of hepatitis C among injecting drug users in England and Wales: is harm reduction working? *American Journal of Public Health*, **91**, 38–42

Horspool MJ, Seivewright N, Armitage CJ & Mathers N (2008). Post-treatment outcomes of buprenorphine detoxification in community settings: a systematic review. *European Addiction Research*, **14**, 179–85

Howells C, Allen S, Gupta J, Stillwell G, Marsden J & Farrell M (2002). Prison based detoxification for opioid dependence: a randomized double blind controlled trial of lofexidine and methadone. *Drug and Alcohol Dependence*, **67**, 169–76

Hubbard RL, Rachal JV, Craddock SG & Cavanagh ER (1984). Treatment Outcome Prospective Study (TOPS): client characteristics and behaviours before, during, and after treatment. In: Timms FM & Ludford JP (eds.) *Drug Abuse Treatment Evaluation: Strategies, Progress and Prospects*. NIDA Research Monograph No. 51

Hubbard RL, Marsden ME, Rachal JV, Harwood HJ, Cavanagh ER & Ginzburg HM (1989). *Drug Abuse Treatment: A National Study of Effectiveness*. University of North Carolina Press

Hughes JR (2007). Smokers who choose to quit gradually versus abruptly. *Addiction*, **102**, 1326–7

Hughes GF, McElnay JC, Hughes CM & McKenna P (1999). Abuse/misuse of non-prescription drugs. *Pharmacy World and Science*, **21**, 251–5

Hughes JR, Stead LF & Lancaster T (2007). Antidepressants for smoking cessation. *Cochrane Database of Systematic Reviews 2007*.

Hulse GK & Basso MR (1999). Reassessing naltrexone maintenance as a treatment for illicit heroin users. *Drug & Alcohol Review*, **18**, 263–9

Hunt GE, Bergen J & Bashir M (2002). Medication compliance and comorbid substance abuse in schizophrenia: impact on community survival 4 years after relapse. *Schizoprenia Research*, **54**, 253–64

Hutchinson SJ, Taylor A, Gruer L, Barr C, Mills C, Elliott L, Goldberg DJ, Scott R & Gilchrist G (2000). One-year follow-up of opiate injectors treated with oral methadone in a GP-centred programme. *Addiction*, **95**, 1055–68

Iguchi MY, Handelsman L, Bickel WK & Griffiths RR (1993). Benzodiazepine and sedative use/abuse by methadone maintenance clients. *Drug and Alcohol Dependence*, **32**, 257–66

Ilgen MA, Jain A, Lucas E & Moos RH (2007). Substance use-disorder treatment and a decline in attempted suicide during and after treatment. *Journal of Studies on Alcohol*, **68**, 303–9

Jaffe JH (2007). Can LAAM, like Lazarus, come back from the dead? *Addiction*, **102**, 1342–3

Jaudes PK, Ekwo E & van Voorhis J (1995). Association of drug abuse and child abuse. *Child Abuse and Neglect*, **19**, 1065–75

Jauffret-Roustide M, Emmanuelli M, Barin F, Arduin P, Laporte A & Desenclos JC (2006). Impact of a harm-reduction policy on HIV and hepatitis C virus transmission among drug users: recent French data—The ANRS-Coquelicot study. *Substance Use and Misuse: An International Interdisciplinary Forum*, **41**, 1603–21

Jenkinson RA, Clark NC, Fry CL & Dobbin M (2005). Buprenorphine diversion and injection in Melbourne, Australia: an emerging issue? *Addiction*, **100**, 197–205

Jerrell JM & Ridgeley MS (1995). Comparative effectiveness of three approaches to serving people with severe mental illness and substance abuse disorders. *Journal of Nervous and Mental Disease*, **183**, 566–76

Johansson BA, Berglund M & Lindgren A (2006). Efficacy of maintenance treatment with naltrexone for opioid dependence: a meta-analytical review. *Addiction*, **101**, 491–503

Johnson S (1997). Dual diagnosis of severe mental illness and substance misuse: a case for specialist services? *British Journal of Psychiatry*, **171**, 205–8

Johnson K, Gerada C & Greenough A (2003). Substance misuse during pregnancy. *British Journal of Psychiatry*, **183**, 187–9

Justo D, Gal-Oz A, Paran Y, Goldin Y & Zeltser D (2006). Methadone-associated Torsades de pointes (polymorphic ventricular tachycardia) in opioid-dependent patients. *Addiction*, **101**, 1333–8

Kakko J, Svanborg KD, Kreek MJ & Heilig M (2003). 1-year retention and social function after buprenorphine-assisted relapse prevention treatment for heroin dependence in Sweden: a randomized, placebo-controlled trial. *Lancet*, **361**, 662–8

Kaminer Y (2002). Adolescent substance abuse treatment: evidence-based practice in outpatient services. *Current Psychiatry Reports*, **4**, 397–401

Kaminer Y, Burleson JA & Goldberger R (2002). Cognitive-behavioral coping skills and psychoeducation therapies for adolescent substance abuse. *Journal of Nervous & Mental Disease*, **190**, 737–45

Kampman KM (2008). The search for medications to treat stimulant dependence. *Addiction Science & Clinical Practice*, **4**, 28–35

Kandel DB & Davies M (1992). Progression to regular marijuana involvement: phenomenology and risk factors for near daily use. In: Glanz M & Pickens R (eds.) *Vulnerability to Drug Abuse*. Washington: American Psychological Association, pp. 211–53

Kantak KM (2003). Anti-cocaine vaccines: antibody protection against relapse. *Expert Opinion Pharmacotherapy*, **4**, 213–8

Kavanagh DJ, White A & Young R (2000). Towards an integrated and sensitive family intervention for comorbid substance abuse and schizophrenia: a comment on Sheils and Rolfe. *Australian Journal of Family Therapy*, **21**, 88–90

Kavanagh DJ, McGrath J, Saunders JB, Dore G & Clark D (2002). Substance misuse in patients with schizophrenia. *Therapy in Practice*, **62**, 743–55

Kaye AD, Gevirtz C, Bosscher HA, Duke JB, Frost EAM, Richards TA & Fields AM (2003). Ultrarapid opiate detoxification: a review. *Canadian Journal of Anesthesia*, **50**, 663–71

Keen J, Oliver P, Rowsse G & Mathers N (2001). Residential rehabilitation for drug users: a review of 13 months' intake to a therapeutic community. *Family Practice*, **18**, 545–8

Keen J, Oliver P, Rowse G & Mathers N (2003). Does methadone maintenance treatment based on the new national guidelines work in a primary care setting? *British Journal of General Practice*, **53**, 461–7

Khan A, Mumford JP, Ash Rogers G & Beckford H (1997). Double-blind study of lofexidine and clonidine in the detoxification of opiate addicts in hospital. *Drug and Alcohol Dependence*, **44**, 57–61

King VL, Kidorf MS, Stoller KB, Carter JA & Brooner RK (2001). Influence of antisocial personality subtypes on drug abuse treatment response. *Journal of Nervous and Mental Disease*, **189**, 593–601

Kintz P (2001). Deaths involving buprenorphine: a compendium of French cases. *Forensic Science International*, **121**, 65–9

Klee H (1992). A new target for behavioural research – amphetamine use. *British Journal of Addiction*, **87**, 439–46

Klee H, Faugier J, Hayes C, Boulton T & Morris J (1990). Aids-related risk behaviour, polydrug use and temazepam. *British Journal of Addiction*, **85**, 1125–32

Klee H, Wright S, Carnwath T & Merrill J (2001). The role of substitute therapy in the treatment of problem amphetamine use. *Drug and Alcohol Review*, **20**, 417–29

Klein GW (1997). Treatment complications of methadone maintenance: the impact of a high dose exogenous opioid on the living skills, learning and cognition of patients. *Alcoholism*, **33**, 55–68

Klingemann HKH (1996). Drug treatment in Switzerland: harm reduction, decentralisation and community response. *Addiction*, **91**, 723–36

Klous MG, Nuijen B, van Den Brink W, van Ree JM & Beijnen JH (2007). Pharmaceutical development of dosage forms of diamorphine for use by heroin addicts. *Pharmaceutisch Weekblad*, **142**, 98–104

Kokkevi A, Stefanis N, Anastasopoulou E & Kostogianni C (1998). Personality disorders in drug abusers: prevalence and their association with AXIS I disorders as predictors of treatment retention. *Addictive Behaviors*, 23, 841–53

Kosten TR, Rounsaville BJ & Kleber HD (1985). Parental alcoholism in opioid addicts. *Journal of Nervous and Mental Disease*, 173, 461–9

Kott A, Habel E & Nottingham W (2001). Analysis of behavioral patterns in five cohorts of patients retained in methadone maintenance programs. *The Mount Sinai Journal of Medicine*, 68, 46–54

Krabbe PF, Koning JPF, Heinen N, Laheij RJF, Victory Van Cauter RM & De Jong CAJ (2003). Rapid detoxification from opioid dependence under general anaesthesia versus standard methadone tapering: abstinence rates and withdrawal distress experiences. *Addiction Biology*, 8, 351–8

Kraus L, Augustin R, Frischer M, Kümmler P, Uhl A & Wiessing L (2003). Estimating prevalence of problem drug use at national level in countries of the European Union and Norway. *Addiction*, 98, 471–85

Krausz M, Verthein U, Degkwitz P, Haasen C & Raschke P (1998). Maintenance treatment of opiate addicts in Germany with medications containing codeine – results of a follow-up study. *Addiction*, 93, 1161–7

Kreek MJ (1978). Medical complications in methadone patients. *Annals of the New York Academy of Sciences*, 311, 110–34

Kreek MJ (2000). Methadone-related opioid agonist pharmacotherapy for heroin addiction. History, recent molecular and neurochemical research and future in mainstream medicine. *Annals of the New York Academy of Sciences*, 909, 186–216

Kristensen I, Lolandsmo T, Isaksen A, Vederhus JK & Clausen T (2006). Treatment of poly-drug-using opiate dependents during withdrawal: towards a standardization on treatment. *BMC Psychiatry*, 6, article 54

Lacroix I, Berrebi C, Chaumerliac M, Lapeyre-Mestre J, Montastruc L & Damase-Michel C (2004). Buprenorphine in pregnant opioid-dependent women: first results of a prospective study. *Addiction*, 99, 209–14

Lader M (1993). Historical development of the concept of tranquillizer dependence. In: Hallstrom C (ed.) *Benzodiazepine Dependence*. Oxford: Oxford Medical Publications, pp. 46–57

Lader M & Morton S (1991). Benzodiazepine problems. *British Journal of Addiction*, 86, 823–8

Langendam MW, Van Brussel GHA, Coutinho RA & van Ameijden EJC (2000). Methadone maintenance cessation of injecting drug use: results from the Amsterdam cohort study. *Addiction*, 95, 591–600

Lavelle T, Hammersley R, Forsyth A & Bain D (1991). The use of buprenorphine and temazepam by drug injectors. *Journal of Addictive Diseases*, 10, 5–14

Leavitt SB, Shinderman M, Maxwell S, Eap CB & Paris P (2000). When 'enough' is not enough: new perspectives on optimal methadone maintenance dose. *Mount Sinai Journal of Medicine*, 67, 404–11

Ledoux S, Miller P, Choquet M & Plant M (2002). Family structure, parent-child relationships, and alcohol and other drug use among teenagers in France and the United Kingdom. *Alcohol and Alcoholism*, 37, 52–60

Lehman AF, Myeers CP, Thompson JW & Corty E (1993). Implications of mental and substance use disorders: a comparison of single and dual diagnosis patients. *Journal of Nervous and Mental Disease*, 181, 365–70

Lenne M, Lintzeris N, Breen C, Harris S, Hawken L, Mattick R & Ritter A (2001). Withdrawal from methadone maintenance treatment: prognosis and participant perspectives. *Australian and New Zealand Journal of Public Health*, 25, 121–5

Levin FR & Lehman AF (1991). Meta-analysis of desipramine as an adjunct in the treatment of cocaine addiction. *Journal of Clinical Psychopharmacology*, 11, 371–8

Ley A, Jeffery JP & McLaren S (2001). Treatment programmes for people with both severe mental illness and substance misuse. *The Cochrane Library*. Chichester, UK: Wiley.

Liappas IA et al. (2003). Zolpidem dependence case series: possible neurobiological mechanisms and clinical management. *Journal of Psychopharmacology*, 17, 131–5

Lile B (2003). Twelve step programs: an update. *Addictive Disorders and their Treatment*, 2, 19–24

Lin SK, Strang J, Su LW, Tsai CJ & Hu WH (1997). Double-blind randomised controlled trial of lofexidine versus clonidine in the treatment of heroin withdrawal. *Drug and Alcohol Dependence*, 48, 127–33

Linehan MM, Dimeff LA, Reynolds SK, Comtois KA, Welch SS, Heagerty P & Kivlahan DR (2002). Dialectal behavior therapy versus comprehensive validation therapy plus 12-step for the treatment of opioid dependent women meeting criteria for borderline personality disorder. *Drug & Alcohol Dependence*, **67**, 13–26

Ling W, Charuvastra C, Collins JF, Barki S, Brown LS, Kintaudi P et al. (1998). Buprenorphine maintenance treatment of opiate dependence: a multicenter, randomized clinical trial. *Addiction*, **93**, 475–86

Lingford-Hughes A & Nutt D (2003). Neurobiology of addiction and implications for treatment. *British Journal of Psychiatry*, **182**, 97–100

Lingford-Hughes AR, Welch S & Nutt DJ (2004). Evidence-based guidelines for the pharmacological management of substance misuse, addiction and comorbidity: recommendations from the British Association for Psychopharmacology. *Journal of Psychopharmacology*, **18**, 293–335

Lintzeris N (2002). Buprenorphine dosing regime in the management of outpatient heroin withdrawal. *Drug and Alcohol Review*, **21**, 39–45

Lintzeris N, Holgate F & Dunlop A (1996). Addressing dependent amphetamine use: A place for prescription. *Drug and Alcohol Review*, **15**, 189–95

Lintzeris N, Bell J, Bammer G, Jolley DJ & Rushworth L (2002). A randomized controlled trial of buprenorphine in the management of short-term ambulatory heroin withdrawal. *Addiction*, **97**, 1395–1404

Lowe E & Shewan D (1999). Patterns of alcohol use among methadone clients in a Glasgow housing estate. *Journal of Psychoactive Drugs*, **31**, 145–54

Lubman DI, Hides L & Yucel M (2006). Inhalant misuse in youth: time for a coordinated response. *Medical Journal of Australia*, **185**, 327–30

Luty J (2003). What works in drug addiction? *Advances in Psychiatric Treatment*, **9**, 280–7

Luty J, O'Gara C & Sessay M (2005). Is methadone too dangerous for opiate addiction? *British Medical Journal*, **331**, 1352–3

MacLeod J, Whittaker A & Robertson JR (1998). Changes in opiate treatment during attendance at a community drug service – findings from a clinical audit. *Drug and Alcohol Review*, **17**, 19–25

Magura S & Rosenblum A (2001). Leaving methadone treatment: lessons learned, lessons forgotten, lessons ignored. *The Mount Sinai Journal of Medicine*, **68**, 62–74

Magura S, Nwakeze PC, Kang SY & Demsky S (1999). Program quality effects on patient outcomes during methadone maintenance: a study of 17 clinics. *Substance Use and Misuse*, **34**, 1299–1324

Man LH, Best D, Gossop M, Stillwell G & Strang J (2004). Relationship between prescribing and risk of opiate overdose among drug users in and out of maintenance treatment. *European Addiction Research*, **10**, 35–40

Mann K, Lehert P & Morgan MY (2004). The efficacy of acamprosate in the maintenance of abstinence in alcohol-dependent individuals: results of meta-analysis. *Alcoholism Clinical and Experimental Research*, **28**, 51–63

Mant A & Walsh RA (1997). Reducing benzodiazepine use. *Drug and Alcohol Review*, **16**, 77–84

Margolese HC, Malchy L, Negrate JC, Tempier R & Gill K (2004). Drug and alcohol use among patients with schizophrenia and related psychoses: levels and consequences. *National Library of Medicine*, **67**, 157–66

Margolin A (2003). Acupuncture for substance abuse. *Clinical Psychiatry Reports*, **5**, 333–9

Markovitz PJ (2004). Recent trends in the pharmacotherapy of personality disorders. *Journal of Personality Disorders,* **18**, 90–101

Marks J, Palombella A & Newcombe R (1991). The smoking option. *Druglink*, May/June, 10–11

Marlatt GA & Gordon JR (eds.) (1985). *Relapse Prevention: Maintenance Strategies in the Treatment of Addictive Behaviours*. New York: Guilford Press

Marsch LA (1998). The efficacy of methadone maintenance interventions in reducing illicit opiate use, HIV risk behaviour and criminality: a meta-analysis. *Addiction*, **93**, 515–32

Marsch LA, Bickel WK, Badger GJ, Stothart ME, Quesnel KJ, Stranger C & Brooklyn J (2005). Comparison of pharmacological treatments for opioid-dependent adolescents: a randomized controlled trial. *Archives of General Psychiatry*, **62**, 1157–64

Martino S, Carroll KM, Nich C & Rounsaville BJ (2006). A randomised controlled pilot study of motivational interviewing for patients with psychotic and drug use disorders. *Addiction*, **101**, 1479–92

Maslin J, Graham H, Cawley M, Copello A, Birchwood M, Georgiou G, McGovern D, Mueser K & Orford J (2001). Combined severe mental health and substance use problems. What are the training and support needs of staff working with this client group? *Journal of Mental Health*, **10**, 131–40

Mason BJ, Kocsis JH, Melia D, Khuri ET, Sweeney J, Wells A, Borg L, Millman RB & Kreek MJ (1998). Psychiatric comorbidity in methadone maintained patients. *Journal of Addictive Disorders*, **17**, 75–89

Matheson C, Pitcairn J, Bond CM, van Teijlingen E & Ryan M (2003). General practice management of illicit drug users in Scotland: a national survey. *Addiction*, **98**, 119–26

Mattick RP, Breen C, Kimber J & Davoli M (2002). Methadone maintenance therapy versus no opioid replacement therapy for opioid dependence. *Cochrane Database Systematic Reviews*, **4**

Mattick RP & Hall W (1996). Are detoxification programmes effective? *Lancet*, **347**, 97–100

Mattick RP, Ali R, White JM, O'Brien S, Walk S & Danz C (2003). Buprenorphine versus methadone maintenance therapy: a randomized double-blind trial with 405 opioid-dependent patients. *Addiction*, **98**, 441–52

Mattick RP, Kimber J, Breen C & Davoli M (2004). Buprenorphine maintenance versus placebo or methadone maintenance for opioid dependence (Cochrane Review). *The Cochrane Library*, issue 2. Chichester, UK: John Wiley & Sons

Mattson ME, Del Boca FK, Carroll KM, Cooney NL, DiClemente CC, Donovan D, Kadden RM, McRee B, Rice C, Rycharik RG & Zweben A (1998). Compliance with treatment and follow-up protocols in project MATCH: predictors and relationship to outcome. *Alcoholism Clinical and Experimental Research*, **22**, 1328–39

Maxwell S & Shinderman MS (2002). Optimizing long-term response to methadone maintenance treatment: a 152-week follow-up using higher-dose methadone. *Journal of Addictive Diseases*, **21**, 1–12

McBride AJ, Sullivan JT & Blewett A (1997). Amphetamine prescribing as a harm reduction measure: a preliminary study. *Addiction Research*, **5**, 95–112

McBride AJ, Pates R, Ramadan R & McGowan C (2003). Delphi survey of experts' opinions on strategies used by community pharmacists to reduce over-the-counter drug misuse. *Addiction*, **98**, 487–97

McCambridge J & Strang J (2005). Deterioration over time in effect of motivational interviewing in reducing drug consumption and related risk among young people. *Addiction*, **100**, 470–8

McCusker M (2001). Influence of hepatitis C status on alcohol consumption in opiate users in treatment. *Addiction*, **96**, 1007–14

McDuff DR, Schwartz RP, Tommasello A, Tiegel S, Conovan T & Johnson JL (1993). Outpatient benzodiazepine detoxification procedure for methadone patients. *Journal of Substance Abuse Treatment*, **10**, 297–302

McGlothin WH & Anglin MD (1981). Long-term follow-up of clients of high- and low-dose methadone programs. *Archives of General Psychiatry*, **38**, 1055–63

McGregor C, Machin A & White JM (2003). In-patient benzodiazepine withdrawal: comparison of fixed and symptom-triggered taper methods. *Drug and Alcohol Review*, **22**, 175–80

McKetin R, McLaren J, Lubman DI & Hides L (2006). The prevalence of psychotic symptoms among methamphetamine users. *Addiction*, **101**, 1473–8

McLellan AT, Childress AR, Ehrman R, O'Brien CP & Pashko S (1986). Extinguishing conditioned responses during opiate dependence treatment: turning laboratory findings into clinical procedures. *Journal of Substance Abuse Treatment*, **3**, 33–40

McLellan AT, Arndt IO, Metzger DS, Woody GE & O'Brien CP (1993). The effects of psychosocial services in substance abuse treatment. *Journal of the American Medical Association*, **269**, 1953–9

McMahon T & Rounsaville BJ (2002). Substance misuse and fathering: adding poppa to the research agenda. *Addiction*, **97**, 1109–15

McNeill A, Raw M, Whybrow J & Bailey P (2005). A national strategy for smoking cessation treatment in England. *Addiction*, **100** (suppl 2), 1–11

Megarbane B, Hreiche R, Pirnay S, Nicolas M & Baud FJ (2006). Does high-dose buprenorphine cause respiratory depression?: possible mechanisms and therapeutic consequences. *Toxicological Reviews*, **25**, 79–85

Menezes PR, Johnson S, Thornicroft G, Marshall J, Prosser D, Bebbington P & Kuipers E (1996). Drug and alcohol problems among individuals with severe mental illness in South London. *British Journal of Psychiatry*, **168**, 612–9

Merrill J & Marshall R (1997). Opioid detoxification using naloxone. *Drug and Alcohol Review*, **16**, 3–6

Merrill J, McBride A, Pates R, Peters L, Tetlow A, Roberts C, Arnold K, Crean J, Lomax S & Deakin B (2005). Dexamphetamine substitution as a treatment of amphetamine dependence: a two-centre randomized controlled trial. *Drugs: Education, Prevention & Policy*, **12**, 94–97

Metrebian N, Shanahan W, Stimson GV et al. (1996). Heroin prescribing in the United Kingdom: an overview. *European Addiction Research*, **2**, 194–200

Metrebian N, Shanahan W, Stimson GV et al. (2001). Prescribing drug of choice to opiate dependent drug users: a comparison of clients receiving heroin with those receiving injectable methadone at a West London drug clinic. *Drug and Alcohol Review*, **20**, 267–76

Metrebian N, Mott J, Carnwath Z, Carnwath T, Stimson GV & Sell L (2007). Pathways into receiving a prescription for diamorphine (heroin) for the treatment of opiate dependence in the United Kingdom. *European Addiction Research*, **13**, 144–7

Metzer DS, Woody GE, McLellan AT, O'Brien CP, Druley P, Navaline H, De Phillipis D, Stolley P & Abrutyn E (1993). Human immunodeficiency virus seroconversion among intravenous drug users in- and out-of-treatment: an eighteen month prospective follow-up. *Journal of the Acquired Immune Deficiency Syndrome*, **6**, 1049–56

Milby JB, Gurwitch RH, Wiebe DJ, Ling W, McLellan AT & Woody GE (1986). Prevalence and diagnostic reliability of methadone maintenance detoxification fear. *American Journal of Psychiatry*, **143**, 739–43

Miller WR & Rollnick S (2002). *Motivational Interviewing: Preparing People for Change*. New York: Guildford Press

Milroy CM, Clark JC & Forrest ARW (1996). Pathology of deaths associated with 'ecstasy' and 'eve' misuse. *Journal of Clinical Pathology*, **49**, 149–53

Mintzer MZ & Stitzer ML (2002). Cognitive impairment in methadone maintenance patients. *Drug and Alcohol Dependence*, **67**, 41–51

Miotto K, McCann M, Basch J, Rawson R & Ling W (2002). Naltrexone and dysphoria: fact or myth? *American Journal of Addictions*, **11**, 151–60

Mitchell TB, White JM, Somogyi AA & Bochner F (2003). Comparative pharmacodynamics and pharmacokinetics of methadone and slow-release oral morphine for maintenance treatment of opioid dependence. *Drug and Alcohol Dependence*, **72**, 85–94

Mitchell TB, White JM, Somogyi AA & Bochner F (2004). Slow-release oral morphine versus methadone: a crossover comparison of patient outcomes and acceptability as maintenance pharmacotherapies for opioid dependence. *Addiction*, **99**, 940–5

Mitka M (2003). Office-based primary care physicians called on to treat the "new" addict. *Journal of the American Medical Association*, **290**, 735–6

Moeller FG, Schmitz JM, Steinberg JL, Green CM, Reist C, Lai LY, Swann AC & Grabowski J (2007). Citalopram combined with behavioral therapy reduces cocaine use: a double-blind, placebo-controlled trial. *American Journal of Drug & Alcohol Abuse*, **33**, 367–78

Moeller KE, Lee KC & Kissack JC (2008). Urine drug screening: practical guide for clinicians. *Mayo Clinic Proceedings*, **83**, 66–76

Moore THM, Zammit S, Lingford-Hughes A & Barnes TRE (2007). Cannabis use and risk of psychotic or affective mental health outcomes: a systematic review. *The Lancet*, **370**, 319–28

Moran P, Coffey C, Mann A, Carlin JB & Patton GC (2006). Personality and substance use disorders in young adults. *The British Journal of Psychiatry*, **188**, 374–9

Morgan CJA & Curran HV (2008). Effects of cannabidiol on schizophrenia-like symptoms in people who use cannabis. *The British Journal of Psychiatry*, **192**, 306–7

Morrison CL & Ruben SM (1995). The development of health care services for drug misusers and prostitutes. *Postgraduate Medical Journal*, **71**, 593–7

Mos J & Oliver B (1987). Pro-aggressive actions of benzodiazepines. In: Oliver B, Mos J & Brain PF (eds.) *Ethopharmacology of Agonistic Behaviour in Animals and*

Humans. Dordrecht: Martinus Nijhoff, pp. 187–206

Mueser KT, Drake RE, Alterman AI & Ackerson TH (1997). Antisocial personality disorder, conduct disorder, and substance abuse in schizophrenia. *Journal of Abnormal Psychology*, **106**, 473–7

Muga R, Sanvisens F, Bolao F, Tor J, Santesmases J, Pujol R, Tural C, Langohr K, Rey-Joly C & Munoz A (2006). Significant reductions in HIV prevalence but not of hepatitis C virus infections in injection drug users from metropolitan Barcelona. *Drug and Alcohol Dependence*, **82**, S29–S33

Mulder RT (2002). Personality pathology and treatment outcome in major depression: a review. *American Journal of Psychiatry*, **159**, 359–71

Musselman DL & Kell MJ (1995). Prevalence and improvement in psychopathology in opioid dependent patients participating in methadone maintenance. *Journal of Addictive Diseases*, **14**, 67–82

Myles J (1997). Treatment for amphetamine use in the United Kingdom. In: Klee H (ed.) *Amphetamine Misuse, International Perspectives on Current Trends.* The Netherlands: Harwood Academic Publishers, pp. 69–79

Myrick H & Brady K (2001). Management of comorbid anxiety and substance use disorders. *Psychiatric Annals*, **31**, 265–71

Myton T & Fletcher K (2003). Descriptive study of the effects of altering formulation of prescribed methadone from injectable to oral. *Psychiatric Bulletin*, **27**, 3–6

Negus SS & Woods JH (1995). Reinforcing effects, discriminative stimulus effects, and physical dependence liability of buprenorphine. In: Cowan A & Lewis JW (eds.) *Buprenorphine: Combatting Drug Abuse with a Unique Opioid.* New York: Wiley-Liss, pp. 71–101

Newman RG & Whitehill WB (1979). Double-blind comparison of methadone and placebo maintenance treatments of narcotic addicts in Hong Kong. *Lancet*, **2**, 485–8

Nielsen S, Dietze P, Lee N, Dunlop A & Taylor D (2007). Concurrent buprenorphine and benzodiazepines use and self-reported opioid toxicity in opioid substitution treatment. *Addiction*, **102**, 616–22

Nnadi CU, Mimiko OA, McCurtis HL & Cadet JL (2005). Neuropsychiatric effects of cocaine use disorders. *Journal of National Medical Association*, **97**, 1504–15

Noonan WC & Moyers TB (1997). Motivational interviewing. *Journal of Substance Misuse*, **2**, 8–16

Novick DM & Kreek MJ (2008). Critical issues in the treatment of hepatitis C virus infection in methadone maintenance patients. *Addiction*, **103**, 905–18

Novick DM, Richman BL, Friendman JM, Friendman JE, Fried C, Wilson JP et al. (1993). The medical status of methadone maintenance patients in treatment for 11–18 years. *Drug and Alcohol Dependence*, **33**, 235–45

O'Brien CP (1996). Recent developments in the pharmacotherapy of substance abuse. *Journal of Consulting and Clinical Psychology*, **64**, 677–86

O'Brien CP (2005). Opiate detoxification: what are the goals? *Addiction*, **100**, 1035

O'Leary Hennessy G, De Menil V & Weiss RD (2003). Psychosocial treatments for cocaine dependence. *Current Psychiatry Report*, **5**, 362–4

Ortner R, Jagsch R, Schindler SD, Primorac A, Fischer G & General Practitioner Addiction Team (2004). Buprenorphine maintenance: office-based treatment with addiction clinic support. *European Addiction Research*, **10**, 105–11

Oude Voshaar RC, Couvee JE, Van Balkom AJLM, Mulder PGH & Zitman FG (2006). Strategies for discontinuing long-term benzodiazepine use. *British Journal of Psychiatry*, **189**, 213–220

Oyefeso A, Ghodse H, Clancy C & Corkery JM (1999). Suicide among drug addicts in the UK. *The British Journal of Psychiatry*, **175**, 277–82

Paris J (1996a). Social factors – mechanisms. In: *Social Factors in the Personality Disorders: A Biopsychosocial Approach to Aetiology and Treatment.* Cambridge: Cambridge University Press, pp. 73–94

Paris J (1996b). Psychological factors. In: *Social Factors in the Personality Disorders: A biopsychosocial approach to aetiology and treatment.* Cambridge: Cambridge University Press, pp. 40–63

Parrott AC (2004). MDMA (3,4-methylenedioxymethamphetamine) or ecstasy: the neuropsychobiological implications of taking it at dances and raves. *Neuropsychobiology*, **50**, 329–35

Pates R, McBride A & Arnold K (2005). Needle fixation. In: Pates R, McBride A & Arnold K (eds.) *Injecting Illicit Drugs*. Oxford: Blackwell

Payne-James JJ, Dean PJ & Keys DW (1994). Drug misusers in police custody: a prospective survey. *Journal of the Royal Society of Medicine*, **87**, 13-4

Payte TJ (2003). Methadone treatment. Safe induction techniques. *Heroin Addiction & Related Clinical Problems*, **6**, 35-42

Pearson G (1996). Drugs and deprivation. *Journal of the Royal Society of Health*, April, 113-6

Penk WE, Flannery RB Jr, Irvin E, Geller J, Fisher W & Hanson MA (2000). Characteristics of substance-abusing persons with schizophrenia: the paradox of the dually diagnosed. *Journal of Addictive Diseases*, **19**, 23-30

Peroutka SJ, Newman H & Harris H (1988). Subjective effects of 3,4-methylene-dioxy-methamphetamine in recreational users. *Neuropsychopharmacology*, **1**, 273-7

Pessione F, Degos F, Marcellin P, Duchatelle V, Njapoum C, Martinot-Peignoux M, Degott C, Valla D, Erlinger S & Rueff B (1998). Effect of alcohol consumption on serum hepatitis C virus RNA and histological lesions in chronic hepatitis C. *Hepatology*, **27**, 1717-22

Petitjean S, Stohler R, Deglon J, Livoti S, Waldvogel D, Uehlinger C & Ladewig D (2001). Double-blind randomized trial of buprenorphine and methadone in opiate dependence. *Drug and Alcohol Dependence*, **62**, 97-104

Petry NM (2006). Contingency management treatments. *British Journal of Psychiatry*, **189**, 97-8

Petursson H & Lader MH (1981). Withdrawal from long-term benzodiazepine treatment. *British Medical Journal*, **238**, 643-5

Philips G, Gossop M & Bradley M (1986). The influence of psychological factors on the opiate withdrawal syndrome. *British Journal of Psychiatry*, **149**, 135-8

Phillips AN, Gazzard BG, Clumeck N, Losso MH & Lundgren JD (2007). When should antiretroviral therapy for HIV be started? *British Medical Journal*, **334**, 76-8

Poikolainen K (2002). Antecedents of substance use in adolescence. *Current Opinion in Psychiatry*, **15**, 241-5

Pollack M, Brotman A & Rosenbaum J (1989). Cocaine abuse treatment. *Comprehensive Psychiatry*, **30**, 31-44

Pollack MH, Penava SA, Bolton E, Worthington JJ, Allen GL, Farach FJ & Otto MW (2002). A novel cognitive-behavioral approach for treatment-resistant drug dependence. *Journal of Substance Abuse Treatment*, **23**, 335-42

Polson RG, Fleming PM & O'Shea JK (1993). Fluoxetine in the treatment of amphetamine dependence. *Human Psychopharmacology*, **8**, 55-8

Poole R & Brabbins C (1996). Drug induced psychosis. *British Journal of Psychiatry*, **168**, 135-8

Pozner CN, Levine M & Zane R (2005). The cardiovascular effects of cocaine. *Journal of Emergency Medicine*, **29**, 173-8

Prendergast M, Podus D, Finney J, Greenwell L & Roll J (2006). Contingency management for treatment of substance use disorders: a meta-analysis. *Addiction*, **101**, 1546-60

Preston KL, Griffiths RR, Stitzer ML, Bigelow GE & Liebson IA (1984). Diazepam and methadone interactions in methadone maintenance. *Clinical Pharmacology and Therapeutics*, **36**, 534-41

Preston KL, Umbricht A & Epstein DH (2000). Methadone dose increase and abstinence reinforcement for treatment of continued heroin use during methadone maintenance. *Archives of General Psychiatry*, **57**, 395-404

Preti A (2007). New developments in the pharmacotherapy of cocaine abuse. *Addiction Biology*, **12**, 133-151

Quang-Cantagrel ND, Wallace MS, Ashar N & Mathews C (2001). Long-term methadone treatment: effect on CD4+ lymphocyte counts and HIV-1 plasma RNA level in patients with HIV infection. *European Journal of Pain*, **5**, 415-20

Raistrick D (1997). Substitute prescribing – social policy or individual treatment? (and why we must make the decision). *Druglink*, March/April, 16-17

Raistrick D, West D, Finnegan O, Thistlethwaite G, Brearley R & Banbery J (2005). A comparison of buprenorphine and lofexidine for community opiate detoxification: results from a randomized controlled trial. *Addiction*, **100**, 1860-7

Rawson RA, McCann MJ, Flammino F, Shoptaw S, Mitto K, Reiber C & Ling W (2006). A comparison of contingency management and cognitive-behavioural approaches for stimulant-dependent individuals. *Addiction*, **101**, 267–74

Regier DA, Farmer ME, Rae DS, Locke BZ, Keith SJ, Judd LL & Goodwin FK (1990). Comorbidity of mental disorders with alcohol and other drug abuse. *Journal of the American Medical Association*, **264**, 2511–18

Reuter P & Pollack H (2006). How much can treatment reduce national drug problems? *Addiction*, **101**, 341–7

Reynaud M, Petit G, Potard D & Courty P (1998). Six deaths linked to concomitant use of buprenorphine and benzodiazepines. *Addiction*, **93**, 1385–92

Rhodes T, Briggs D, Kimber J, Jones S & Holloway G (2007). Crack-heroin speedball injection and its implications for vein care: qualitative study. *Addiction*, **102**, 1782–90

Ridenour TA (2005). Inhalants: not to be taken lightly anymore. *Current Opinion in Psychiatry*, **18**, 243–7

Robertson JR, Raab GM, Bruce M, McKenzie JS, Storkey HR & Salter A (2006). Addressing the efficacy of dihydrocodeine versus methadone as an alternative maintenance treatment for opiate dependence: a randomized controlled trial. *Addiction*, **101**, 1752–9

Robson P & Bruce M (1997). A comparison of 'visible' and 'invisible' users of amphetamine, cocaine and heroin: two distinct populations? *Addiction*, **92**, 1729–36

Rodger A, Roberts S, Lanigan A et al. (2000). Assessment of long-term outcomes of community-acquired hepatitis C infection in a cohort with sera stored from 1971 to 1975. *Hepatology*, **32**, 582–7

Rohsenow DJ, Monti PM, Martin RA, Colby SM, Myers MG, Gulliver SB, Brown RA, Mueller TI, Gordon A & Abrams DB (2004). Motivational enhancement and coping skills training for cocaine abusers: effects on substance use outcomes. *Addiction*, **99**, 862–74

Rosen M & Kosten TR (1995). Detoxification and induction onto naltrexone. In: Cowan A & Lewis JW (eds.) *Buprenorphine: Combatting Drug Abuse with a Unique Opioid.* New York: Wiley-Liss, pp. 289–305

Rosenbaum M (1995). The demedicalization of methadone maintenance. *Journal of Psychoactive Drugs*, **27**, 145–9

Rosenbaum M & Murphy S (1984). Always a junkie?: The arduous task of getting off methadone maintenance. *Journal of Drug Issues*, **14**, 527–52

Ross J, Darke S & Hall W (1997). Transitions between routes of benzodiazepine administration among heroin users in Sydney. *Addiction*, **92**, 697–705

Ross J & Darke S (2000). The nature of benzodiazepine dependence among heroin users in Sydney, Australia. *Addiction*, **95**, 1785–93

Rostami-Hodjegan A, Wolff K, Hay AWM, Raistrick D, Calvert R & Tucker GT (1999). Population pharmacokinetics in opiate users: characterization of time dependent changes. *British Journal of Clinical Pharmacology*, **47**, 974–86

Rothman RB & Baumann MH (2006). Balance between dopamine and serotonin release modulates behavioral effects of amphetamine-type drugs. *Annals of the New York Academy of Sciences*, **1074**, 245–60

Rounsaville BJ, Glazer W, Wilber CH, Weissman MM & Kleber HD (1983). Short-term interpersonal psychotherapy in methadone-maintained opiate addicts. *Archives of General Psychiatry*, **40**, 629–36

Rounsaville B, Kosten TR & Kleber HD (1986). Long-term changes in current psychiatric diagnoses of treated opiate addicts. *Comprehensive Psychiatry*, **27**, 489–98

Rowan-Szal GA, Bartholomew NG, Chatham LR & Simpson DD (2005). A combined cognitive and behavioral intervention for cocaine-using methadone clients. *Journal of Psychoactive Drugs*, **37**, 75–84

Ruben SM & Morrison CL (1992). Temazepam misuse in a group of injecting drug users. *British Journal of Addiction*, **87**, 1387–92

Ruben SM, McLean PC & Melville J (1989). Cyclizine abuse among a group of opiate dependents receiving methadone. *British Journal of Addiction*, **84**, 929–34

Rumball D & Williams J (1997). Rapid opiate detoxification. *British Medical Journal*, **315**, 682

Ryder D, Kraszlan K, Lien D, Allen E, Chiplin T, Dick S & Petsos S (2001). The western Australian court Diversion Service: client profile and predictors of program completion, sentencing and re-offending. *Psychiatry Psychology and Law*, **8**, 65–75

Salazar C (1997). Relapse prevention and nursing interventions. In: Rassool GH & Gafoor M (eds.) *Addiction Nursing. Perspectives on Professional and Clinical Practice*. Gloucester: Stanley Thornes, pp. 67–79

San L, Cami J, Peri JM, Mata R & Porta M (1990). Efficacy of clonidine, guanfacine and methadone in the rapid detoxification of heroin addicts: a controlled clinical trial. *British Journal of Addiction*, **85**, 141–7

San L, Pomarol G, Peri JM, Olle JM & Cami J (1991). Follow-up after a six-month maintenance period of naltrexone versus placebo in heroin addicts. *British Journal of Addiction*, **86**, 983–90

San L, Fernandez T, Cami J & Gossop M (1994). Efficacy of methadone versus methadone and guanfacine in the detoxification of heroin-addicted patients. *Journal of Substance Abuse Treatment*, **11**, 463–9

Sarfraz A & Alcorn RJ (1999). Injectable methadone prescribing in the United Kingdom – current practice and future policy guidelines. *Substance Use and Misuse*, **34**, 1709–21

Saunders B, Wilkinson C & Phillips M (1995). The impact of a brief motivational intervention with opiate users attending a methadone programme. *Addiction*, **90**, 415–24

Saxon AJ, Wells EA, Fleming C, Jackson TR & Calsyn DA (1996). Pre-treatment characteristics, program philosophy and level of ancillary services as predictors of methadone maintenance treatment outcome. *Addiction*, **91**, 1197–1209

Schaefer M, Heinz A & Backmund M (2004). Treatment of chronic hepatitis C in patients with drug dependence: time to change the rules? *Addiction*, **99**, 1167–75

Schmittner J, Schroeder JR, Epstein DH & Preston KL (2005). Menstrual cycle length during methadone maintenance. *Addiction*, **100**, 829–36

Schottenfeld RS, Chawarski MC, Pakes JR, Pantalon MV, Carroll KM & Kosten TR (2005). Methadone versus buprenorphine with contingency management or performance feedback for cocaine and opioid dependence. *American Journal of Psychiatry*, **162**, 340–9

Scott H, Johnson S, Menezes P, Thornicroft G, Marshall J, Bindman J et al. (1998). Substance misuse and risk of aggression and offending among the severely mentally ill. *British Journal of Psychiatry*, **172**, 345–50

Scott R (1990). The prevention of convulsions during benzodiazepine withdrawals. *British Journal of General Practice*, **40**, 261

Seifert J, Metzner C, Paetzold W, Borsutzky M, Ohlmeier M, Passie T, Hauser U, Becker H, Wiese B, Emrich HM & Schneider U (2005). Mood and affect during detoxification of opiate addicts: a comparison of buprenorphine versus methadone. *Addiction Biology*, **10**, 157–64

Seivewright N (1998). Theory and practice in managing benzodiazepine dependence and abuse. *Journal of Substance Misuse*, **3**, 170–7

Seivewright N & Daly C (1997). Personality disorder and drug use: a review. *Drug and Alcohol Review*, **16**, 235–50

Seivewright N & Dougal W (1993). Withdrawal symptoms from high dose benzodiazepines in poly drug users. *Drug and Alcohol Dependence*, **32**, 15–23

Seivewright N & Iqbal M (2002). Prescribing to drug misusers in practice – often effective, but rarely straightforward. *Addiction Biology*, **7**, 269–77

Seivewright N & Lagundoye O (2007). What the clinician needs to know about magic mushrooms. In: Day E (ed.) *Clinical Topics in Addiction*. London: RCPsych Publications, pp. 55–9

Seivewright N, Donmall M, Douglas J, Draycott T & Millar T (2000a). Cocaine misuse treatment in England. *International Journal of Drug Policy*, **11**, 203–15

Seivewright N, Tyrer P, Ferguson B, Murphy S & Johnson T (2000b). Longitudinal study of the influence of life events and personality status on diagnostic change in three neurotic disorders. *Depression and Anxiety*, **11**, 105–13

Seivewright N, McMahon C & Egleston P (2005). Stimulant use still going strong. *Advances in Psychiatric Treatment*, **11**, 262–9

Seivewright N, Horsley L & Gadsby K (2006). Additional drug use on methadone programmes – often cocaine rather than heroin. *Psychiatric Bulletin*, **30**, 395

Sell L (2003). Prescribing injectable methadone: to whom and for what purpose? In: Tober G & Strang J (eds.) *Methadone Matters: Evolving Community Methadone Treatment of Methadone Treatment of Opiate Addiction.* London: Martin Dunitz, pp. 107–18

Sell L, Farrell M & Robson P (1997). Prescription of diamorphine, dipipanone and cocaine in England and Wales. *Drug and Alcohol Review*, **16**, 221–6

Sell L, Segar G & Merrill J (2001). One hundred and twenty-five patients prescribed injectable opiates in the North West of England. *Drug and Alcohol Review*, **20**, 57–66

Senay EC, Barthwell AG, Marks R, Bokes P, Gillman D & White R (1993). Medical maintenance: a pilot study. *Journal of Addictive Diseases*, **12**, 59–75

Seow SW, Swensen G, Willis D, Hartfield M & Chapman C (1980). Extraneous drug use in methadone-supported patients. *Medical Journal of Australia*, **1**, 269–71

Shearer J, Wodak A, Mattick RP, van Beek I, Lewis J, Hall W & Dolan K (2001). Pilot randomized controlled study of dexamphetamine substitution for amphetamine dependence. *Addiction*, **96**, 1289–96

Shearer J, Wodak A, van Beek I, Mattick RP & Lewis J (2003). Pilot randomized double blind placebo-controlled study of dexamphetamine for cocaine dependence. *Addiction*, **96**, 1289–96.

Sherman JP (1990). Dexamphetamine for 'speed' addiction. *Medical Journal of Australia*, **153**, 306

Simoens S, Matheson C, Bond C, Inkster K & Ludbrook A (2005). The effectiveness of community maintenance with methadone or buprenorphine for treating opiate dependence. *British Journal of General Practice*, **55**, 139–46

Smith N (2005). High potency cannabis: the forgotten variable. *Addiction*, **100**, 1558–9

Soar K, Turner JJD & Parrott AC (2001). Psychiatric disorders in ecstasy (MDMA) users: a literature review focusing on personal predisposition and drug history. *Human Psychopharmacology: Clinical and Experimental*, **16**, 641–5

Soar K, Parrott AC & Fox HC (2004). Persistent neuropsychological problems after 7 years of abstinence from recreational ecstasy (MDMA): a case study. *Psychological Reports*, **95**, 192–6

Soares B, Limas M, Reisser A & Farrell M (2003). Dopamine agonists for cocaine dependence (Cochrane Review). *The Cochrane Library*. Chichester: John Wiley & Sons

Solberg U, Burkhart G & Nilson M (2002). An overview of opiate substitution treatment in the European Union and Norway. *International Journal of Drug Policy*, **13**, 477–84

Soyka M (2000). Substance misuse, psychiatric disorder and violent and disturbed behaviour. *British Journal of Psychiatry*, **176**, 345–50

Spataro J, Mullen PE, Burgess PM, Wells DL & Moss SA (2004). Impact of child sexual abuse on mental health. Prospective study in males and females. *British Journal of Psychiatry*, **184**, 416–21

Staiger P, Kambouropoulos N & Dawe S (2007). Should personality traits be considered when refining substance misuse treatment programs? *Drug and Alcohol Review*, **26**, 17–23

Stark K, Muller K, Bienzle U & Guggenmoos-Holzmann I (1996). Methadone maintenance treatment and HIV risk-taking behaviour among injecting drug users in Berlin. *Journal of Epidemiology and Community Health*, **50**, 534–7

Steels MD, Hamilton M & McLean PC (1992). The consequences of a change in formulation of methadone prescribed in a drug clinic. *British Journal of Addiction*, **87**, 1549–54

Steinberg KL, Roffman RA, Carroll KM, Kabela E, Kadden R, Miller M & Duresky D (2002). Tailoring cannabis dependence treatment for a diverse population. *Addiction*, **97**, 135–42

Stella L, Cassese F, Barone S, Barchetta A, Iacobelli M, Motola G, Mazzeo F & Rossi F (1999). Naltrexone to keep a drug-free condition. *Research Communications in Alcohol and Substances of Abuse*, **20**, 91–8

Stephens RS, Roffman RA & Curtin L (2000). Comparison of extended versus brief treatments for marijuana use. *Journal of Consulting and Clinical Psychology*, **68**, 898–908

Stephens RS, Roffman RA, Copeland J & Swift W (2006). Cognitive-behavioral and motivational enhancement treatments for cannabis dependence. In: RA Roffman & RS Stephens (eds.) *Cannabis Dependence: Its Nature, Consequences and Treatment*. London: Cambridge University Press, pp. 131–53

Stitzer ML, Griffiths RR, McLellan AT, Graboswki J & Hawthorne JW (1981). Diazepam use among methadone patients: patterns and dosages. *Drug and Alcohol Dependence*, **8**, 189–99

Stitzer ML, Bigelow GE, Liebson IA & Hawthorne JW (1982). Contingent reinforcement for benzodiazepine-free urines: evaluation of a drug abuse treatment intervention. *Journal of Applied Behavioural Analysis*, **15**, 493–503

Strang J & Gossop M (eds.) (1994). *Heroin Addiction and Drug Policy: The British System*. Oxford: Oxford University Press

Strang J & Sheridan J (1997a). Heroin prescribing in the 'British System' of the mid 1990s: data from the 1995 national survey of community pharmacies in England and Wales. *Drug and Alcohol Review*, **16**, 7–16

Strang J & Sheridan J (1997b). Prescribing amphetamines to drug misusers: data from the 1995 National Survey of Community Pharmacies in England & Wales. *Addiction*, **92**, 833–8

Strang J, Donmall M, Webster A & Tantam D (1991). Comparison between community drug teams with and without inbuilt medical services. *British Medical Journal*, **303**, 897

Strang J, Smith M & Spurrell S (1992). The community drug team. *British Journal of Addiction*, **87**, 169–78

Strang J, Sheridan J & Barber N (1996). Prescribing injectable and oral methadone to opiate addicts: results from the 1995 national postal survey of community pharmacies in England and Wales. *British Medical Journal*, **313**, 270–2

Strang J, Marks I, Dawe S, Powell J, Gossop M, Richards D & Gray J (1997). Type of hospital setting and treatment outcome with heroin addicts. Results from a randomised trial. *British Journal of Psychiatry*, **171**, 335–9

Strang J, Marsden J, Cummins M, Farrell M, Finch E, Gossop M, Stewart D & Welch S (2000). Randomized trial of supervised injectable versus oral methadone maintenance: report of feasibility and 6-month outcome. *Addiction*, **95**, 1631–45

Strang J, McCambridge J, Platts S & Groves P (2004). Engaging the reluctant GP in care of the opiate misuser. *Family Practice*, **21**, 150–4

Strang J, Kelleher M, Best D, Mayet S & Manning V (2006). Emergency naloxone for heroin overdose. *British Medical Journal*, **333**, 614–5

Strang J, Hunt C, Gerada C & Marsden J (2007a). What difference does training make? A randomized trial with waiting-list control of general practitioners seeking advanced training in drug misuse. *Addiction*, **102**, 1637–47

Strang J, Manning V, Mayet S, Ridge G, Best D & Sheridan J (2007b). Does prescribing for opiate addiction change after national guidelines? Methadone and buprenorphine prescribing to opiate addicts by general practitioners and hospital doctors in England, 1995–2005. *Addiction*, **102**, 761–70

Strecher VJ, Shiffman S & West R (2005). Randomized controlled trial of a web-based computer-tailored smoking cessation program as a supplement to nicotine patch therapy. *Addiction*, **100**, 682–8

Sullivan MA & Covey LS (2002). Current perspectives on smoking cessation among substance abusers. *Current Psychiatry Reports*, **4**, 388–96

Sullivan LE, Metzger DS, Fudala PJ & Fiellin DA (2005). Decreasing international HIV transmission: the role of expanding access to opioid agonist therapies for injection drug users. *Addiction*, **100**, 150–8

Swofford CD, Kasckow JW, Scheller-Gilkey G & Inderbitzin LB (1996). Substance use: a powerful predictor of relapse in schizophrenia. *Schizophrenia Research*, **20**, 145–51

Taikato M, Kidd B & Baldacchino A (2005). What every psychiatrist should know about buprenorphine in substance misuse. *Psychiatric Bulletin*, **29**, 225–7

Tassiopoulos K, Bernstein J, Heeren T, Levenson S, Hingson R & Bernstein E (2004). Hair testing and self-report of cocaine use by heroin users. *Addiction*, **99**, 590–7

Teesson M, Ross J, Darke S, Lynskey M, Ali R, Ritter A & Cooke R (2006). One year outcomes for heroin dependence: findings from the Australian Treatment Outcome Study (ATOS). *Drug and Alcohol Dependence*, **83**, 174–80

Tetlow VA & Merrill J (1996). Rapid determination of amphetamine stereoisomer ratios in urine by gas chromatography–mass spectroscopy. *Annals of Clinical Biochemistry*, **33**, 50–4

Thomasius R, Petersen KU, Zapletalova P, Wartberg L, Zeichner D & Schmoldt A

(2003). Mood, cognition, and serotonin transporter availability in current and former ecstasy (MDMA) users. *Psychopharmacology*, **167**, 85–96

Thomasius R, Petersen KU, Zapletalova P, Wartberg L, Zeichner D & Schmoldt A (2005). Mental disorders in current and former heavy ecstasy (MDMA) users. *Addiction*, **100**, 1310–9

Tiet QQ, Ilgen MA, Byrnes HF & Moos RH (2006). Suicide attempts among substance use disorder patients: an initial step towards a decision tree for suicide management. *Alcoholism: Clinical and Experimental Research*, **30**, 998–1005

Tremeau F, Darreye A, Leroy B, Renckly V, Ertle S, Weibel H, Khidichian F & Macher JP (2003). Personality changes in opioid-dependent subjects in a methadone maintenance treatment program. *L'Encephale*, **29**, 285–92

Tretter F, Burkhardt D, Bussello-Spieth B, Reiss J, Walcher S & Buchele W (1998). Clinical experience with antagonist-induced opiate withdrawal under anaesthesia. *Addiction*, **93**, 269–75

Troisi A, Pasini A, Saracco M & Spalletta G (1998). Psychiatric symptoms in male cannabis users not using other illicit drugs. *Addiction*, **93**, 487–92

Tyrer P & Weaver T (2004). Desperately seeking solutions: the search for appropriate treatment for comorbid substance misuse and psychosis. *Psychiatric Bulletin*, **28**, 1–2

Tyrer P, Rutherford D & Huggett T (1981). Benzodiazepine withdrawal symptoms and propranolol. *Lancet*, **i**, 520–2

Tyrer P, Seivewright N, Ferguson B, Murphy S, Darling C, Brothwell J et al. (1990). The Nottingham Study of Neurotic Disorder: relationship between personality status and symptoms. *Psychological Medicine*, **20**, 423–31

Uchtenhagen A, Dobler-Mikola A & Gutzwiller (1996). Medical prescriptions of narcotics. *European Addiction Research*, **2**, 201–7

van Ameijden EJC, Langendem MW & Coutinho RA (1999). Dose-effect relationship between overdose mortality and prescribed methadone dosage in low-threshold maintenance programs. *Addictive Behaviours*, **24**, 559–63

van de Laar MC, Licht R, Franken IHA & Hendricks VM (2004). Event-related potentials indicate motivational relevance of cocaine use in abstinent cocaine addicts. *Psychopharmacology*, **177**, 121–9

Van den Berg C, Smit C, van Brussel G, Coutinho R & Prins M (2007). Full participation in harm reduction programmes is associated with decreased risk for human immunodeficiency virus and hepatitis C virus: evidence from the Amsterdam Cohort Studies amoung drug users. *Addiction*, **102**, 1454–62

van den Bosch LMC & Verheul R (2007). Patients with addiction and personality disorder: treatment outcomes and clinical implications. *Current Opinion in Psychiatry*, **20**, 67–71

van den Brink W, Hendriks VM, Blanken P, Koeter MWJ, van Zwieten BJ & van Ree JM (2003). Medical prescription of heroin to treatment resistant heroin addicts: two randomized controlled trials. *British Medical Journal*, **327**, 310–2

van Valkenburg C & Akiskal H (1999). Which patients presenting with clinical anxiety will abuse benzodiazepines? *Human Psychopharmacology*, **14**, 45–51

Vaughan EL & McMahon RC (2006). Changes over time in addiction severity index problem dimensions among cocaine abusers treated in community settings. *Substance Use and Misuse*, **41**, 1287–94

Vecellio M, Schopper C & Modestin J (2003). Neuropsychiatric consequences (atypical psychosis and complex-partial seizures) of ecstasy use: possible evidence for toxicity-vulnerability predictors and implications for preventative and clinical care. *Journal of Psychopharmacology*, **17**, 342–5

Verdoux H (2004). Cannabis and psychosis proneness. In: Castle D & Murray R (eds.) *Marijuana and Madness: Psychiatry and Neurobiology*. Cambridge: Cambridge University Press, pp. 75–88

Verheul R, van den Brink W & Hartgers C (1995). Prevalence of personality disorders among alcoholics and drug addicts: an overview. *European Addiction Research*, **1**, 166–77

Vignau J & Brunelle E (1998). Differences between general practitioner- and addiction centre-prescribed buprenorphine substitution therapy in France. Preliminary results. *European Addiction Research*, **4**, suppl 1, 24–8

Vocci FJ & Appel NM (2007). Approaches to the development of medications for the treatment of methamphetamine dependence. *Addiction*, **102** (suppl 1), 96–106

Volkow ND & Li TK (2004). Drug addiction: The neurobiology of behaviour gone awry. *Nature Reviews Neuroscience*, **5**, 963–70

Vorma H, Naukkarinen H, Sarna S & Kuoppa-salmi K (2002). Treatment of out-patients with complicated benzodiazepine dependence: comparison of two approaches. *Addiction*, **97**, 851–9

Wagner AF & Anthony JC (2002). Into the world of illegal drug use: exposure opportunity and other mechanisms linking the use of alcohol, tobacco, marijuana and cocaine. *American Journal of Epidemiology*, **155**, 918–25

Walker R (1992a). Substance abuse and B-cluster disorders. I: Understanding the dual diagnosis patient. *Journal of Psychoactive Drugs*, **24**, 223–32

Walker R (1992b). Substance abuse and B-cluster disorders. II: Treatment recommendations. *Journal of Psychoactive Drugs*, **24**, 233–41

Walsh SL & Eissenberg T (2003). The clinical pharmacology of buprenorphine: extrapolating from the laboratory to the clinic. *Drug & Alcohol Dependence*, **70**, suppl 13–27

Walsh SL, Preston KL, Stitzer ML, Cone EJ & Bigelow GE (1994). Clinical pharmacology of buprenorphine: ceiling effects at high doses. *Clinical Pharmacology and Therapeutics*, **55**, 569–80

Walsh SL, Strain EC & Bigelow GE (2003). Evaluation of the effects of lofexidine and clonidine on naloxone-precipitated withdrawal in opioid-dependent humans. *Addiction*, **98**, 427–39

Ward J, Mattick RP & Hall W (1998a). *Methadone Maintenance Treatment and Other Opioid Replacement Therapies.* London: Harwood

Ward J, Mattick RP & Hall W (1998b). How long is long enough? Answers to questions about the duration of methadone maintenance treatment. In: Ward J, Mattick RP & Hall W (eds.) *Methadone Maintenance Treatment and Other Opioid Replacement Therapies.* London: Harwood, pp. 305–36

Ward J, Hall W & Mattick RP (1999). Role of maintenance treatment in opioid dependence. *Lancet*, **353**, 221–6

Weaver T, Madden P, Charles V, Stimson G, Renton A, Tyrer P, Barnes T, Bench C, Middleton H, Wright N, Paterson S,

Shanahan W, Seivewright N & Ford C (2003). Comorbidity of substance misuse and mental illness in community mental health and substance misuse services. *British Journal of Psychiatry*, **183**, 304–13

Webster LR (2005). Methadone-related deaths. *Journal of Opioid Management*, **1**, 211–7

Weiss RD, Griffin ML, Gallop RJ, Najavits LM, Arlene F, Crits-Christoph P, Thase ME, Blaine J, Gastfriend DR, Daley D & Luborsky L (2005). The effect of 12-step self-help group attendance and participation on drug use outcomes among cocaine-dependent patients. *Drug and Alcohol Dependence*, **77**, 177–84

Weizman T, Gelkopf M, Melamed Y, Adelson M & Beleich A (2003). Treatment of benzodiazepine dependence in methadone maintenance treatment patients: a comparison of two therapeutic modalities and the role of psychiatric comorbidity. *Australian and New Zealand Journal of Psychiatry*, **37**, 458–63

Welch S (2007). Substance use and personality disorders. *Psychiatry*, **6**, 27–9

West R, McEwen A, Bolling K & Owen L (2001). Smoking cessation and smoking patterns in the general population. *Addiction*, **96**, 891–902

Westermeyer J (1995). Cultural aspects of substance abuse and alcoholism. *Psychiatric Clinics of North America*, **18**, 589–605

Widiger TA, Simonsen E, Krueger R, Livesley WJ & Verheul R (2005). Personality disorder research agenda for the DSM-V. *Journal of Personality Disorders*, **19**, 215–38

Williams H, Oyefeso A & Ghodse AH (1996). Benzodiazepine misuse and dependence among opiate addicts in treatment. *Irish Journal of Psychological Medicine*, **13**, 62–4

Williams H, Handyside D, Bashford K & Oyefeso A (2005). Service response to benzodiazepine use in opiate addicts: a national postal survey. *Irish Journal of Psychological Medicine*, **22**, 15–8

Williamson A, Darke S, Ross J & Teesson M (2006). The association between cocaine use and short-term outcomes for the treatment of heroin dependence: findings from the Australian Treatment Outcome Study (ATOS). *Drug and Alcohol Review*, **25**, 141–8

Withers NW, Pulvirenti L, Koob GF & Gillin JC (1995). Cocaine abuse and dependence. *Journal of Clinical Psychopharmacology*, **15**, 63–78

Wodak A (1994). Managing illicit drug use: a practical guide. *Drugs*, **47**, 446–57

Wodak A (1997). Hepatitis C: waiting for the Grim Reaper. *Medical Journal of Australia*, **166**, 290–3

Wodak A, Seivewright NA, Wells B, Reuter P, Des Jarlais DC, Rezza G et al. (1994). Comments on: Ball & van de Wijngaart's 'A Dutch addict's view on methadone maintenance – an American and a Dutch appraisal'. *Addiction*, **89**, 803–14

Wolff K (2002). Characterization of methadone overdose: clinical considerations and the scientific evidence. *Theraputic Drug Monitoring*, **24**, 457–70

Worm K, Steentoft A & Kringsholm B (1993). Methadone and drug addicts. *International Journal of Legal Medicine*, **106**, 119–23

Yancovitz SR, Des Jarlais DC, Peyser NP, Drew E, Freidmann P, Trigg HL & Robinson JW (1991). A randomised trial of an interim methadone maintenance clinic. *American Journal of Public Health*, **81**, 1185–91

Zammit S, Allebeck P, Andreasson S, Lundberg I & Lewis G (2002). Self reported cannabis use as a risk factor for schizophrenia in Swedish conscripts of 1969: historical cohort study. *British Medical Journal*, **325**, 1195–1212

Zhang Z, Friedman PD & Gersteine DR (2003). Does retention matter? Treatment duration and improvement in drug use. *Addiction*, **98**, 673–84

Index